Contents

Break the Sugar Habit 2

The Important Sugars 2

A very new and deadly addition to our diet 3

How to tell if you're addicted to sugar 4

Avoiding Fructose 5

Getting Fructose Out of Your Diet 5

Sugar Substitutes 7

Seed Oils 8

The Lists 9

More Information 188

Break the Sugar Habit

Governments spend a fortune on programs aimed at making us lose weight. They tell us to eat less fatty food and exercise more. Meanwhile we fork over ever-increasing amounts on gym memberships, packaged meals, books, magazines and the advice of experts. Despite decades of this we are now fatter than at any other time in history.

Increasingly the signs are that sugar, or more specifically, fructose (the sugar in fruit, and one half of table sugar), is the culprit behind the obesity crisis.

The Important Sugars

There are only three important simple sugars: glucose, fructose and galactose. All of the other sugars you are likely to encounter in daily life are simply combinations of these three.

Glucose is by far the most plentiful of the simple sugars. Pretty much every food (except meat) contains significant quantities of glucose. Even meat (protein) is eventually converted to glucose by our digestive system. It's a pretty important sugar to humans, as it is our primary fuel – no glucose means no us.

Galactose is present in our environment in only very small quantities and is found mainly in dairy products in the form of lactose (where it is joined to a glucose molecule).

Fructose is also relatively rare in nature. It is found primarily in ripe fruits, which is why it is sometimes call fruit sugar. It is usually found together with glucose and it is what makes food taste sweet. As well as fruit, it's naturally present in honey (40%), Maple Syrup (35%) and Agave Syrup (90%).

Sucrose is what we think of when someone says table sugar. It's one half glucose and one half fructose. Brown sugar, caster sugar, raw sugar and Low GI sugar are all just sucrose.

High Fructose Corn Syrup (HFCS) is also approximately one half glucose and one half fructose, just like sucrose. HFCS is just sugar made from corn rather than grass (sugar cane) or beets and it is biochemically identical to those sugars. Throughout this book I just refer to the 'Sugar' content of a product. In doing so, I am including the HFCS as well.

A very new and deadly addition to our diet

In 1822, the only way you could eat a significant amount of sugar (and therefore fructose) was to be the king of England or to come into the small fortune required to buy sugar or honey. We now eat in a month what the average person in 1822 ate in 1 year and 4 months.

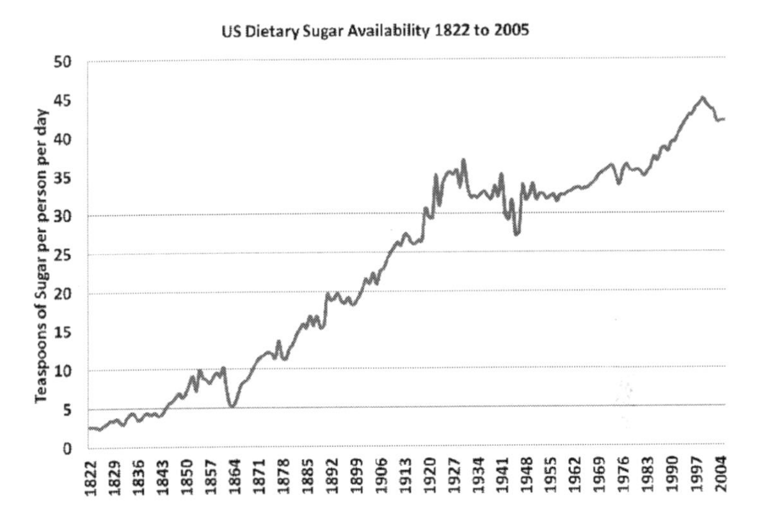

Soft-drink and fruit juice consumption alone has increased by 30 percent in just the last two decades and two thirds of the adult population is now overweight or obese. Today our collective weight problem continues to accelerate in direct proportion to our consumption of sugar.

A slew of recent research makes it clear that as a species we are ill-equipped to deal with the relatively large amounts of sugar (and therefore fructose) we now consume.

The research shows we have one primary appetite-control centre in our brain called the hypothalamus. It reacts to four major appetite hormones. Three of these hormones tell us when we have had enough to eat and one of them temporarily inhibits the effect of the other three and tells us that we need to eat.

Fructose, uniquely among the food we eat, will not stimulate the release of any of the 'enough to eat' hormones. So we can eat it (and any food containing it) without feeling full. Worse still, fructose is not used for energy by our bodies. Instead all of the fructose is directly converted to fat by our livers. This means that by the time we finish our glass of apple juice (or cola or chocolate bar) the first mouthful will already be circulating in our bloodstream as fat.

Just to put the icing on the cake, recent research has now confirmed what most chocolate lovers have always suspected – sugar is as addictive as cocaine.

How to tell if you're addicted to sugar

Do you struggle to walk past a sugary treat without taking 'just one'?

Do you have routines around sugar consumption – for example, always having pudding or needing a piece of chocolate to relax in front of the TV or treating yourself to a sweet drink or chocolate after a session at the gym?

Are there are times when you feel as if you cannot go on without a sugar hit?

If you are forced to go without sugar for 24 hours, do you develop headaches and mood swings?

Obesity is just symptom of a litany of diseases caused by our fructose addiction. Some diseases are directly related to increased body weight, such as osteoarthritis, fractures , hernia and sleep apnoea. Some are related to the way in which fructose messes with our hormones, such as acne and polycystic ovary syndrome. Others are caused by the fructose induced flood of blood-borne fatty acids, notably cardiovascular diseases, fatty liver disease and type II diabetes. And recent research is also suggesting our overindulgence in fructose is directly linked to a variety of cancers, chronic kidney disease, erectile dysfunction and Alzheimer's disease.

Avoiding Fructose

The addictive ingredient in sugar is the fructose. And because it is addictive, food manufacturers have included it in just about everything.

Getting Fructose Out of Your Diet

Breaking a sugar addiction means that before you even start you've got to pick your way through a minefield of fructose filled foods. But in every category of foods there are some which are much lower in fructose than others. This Guide is all about helping you find those low fructose foods.

We know how difficult it is to stop smoking. Imagine how hard it would be if everything we ate or drank contained nicotine. Because much of our food is laced with fructose, breaking a sugar habit is far harder than giving up smoking. But if you use this guide to help with the shopping, you will have avoided most dietary fructose.

The rules for including a food are pretty simple:

1. **Drinks must have no fructose per 100ml.**
2. **Foods must have less than 1.5g of fructose per 100g (less than 3g per 100g of 'Sugars' on the label)**

The reason for the harsh limit on drinks is that we usually drink much more than 100 ml at a time. A can of soft drink is 12 oz (355 ml), a bottle is 20 oz (592 ml) and some fast food outlets serve soft drink in 32 oz (946 ml) sizes. Foods on the other hand are often served at or around the hundred gram mark (except yogurts and ice-creams which are usually 6 oz or 8 oz – 175 ml or 237 ml).

The label on the food is the primary source for information about fructose content. "Sugars" on the label are assumed to be sucrose (glucose + fructose) unless the ingredients list indicates otherwise. For example, dairy foods will often contain considerable quantities of lactose (galactose + glucose) which will appear under the heading 'Sugars'. Those foods have the probable lactose content deducted from the sugar's total before fructose content is calculated.

If a food is not in this list then it is either too high in fructose or I am not aware of it (please send me an email david@davidgillespie.org) to let me know about any missing foods.

Only processed foods are included in the list. If you plan to eat whole food only, then you don't need to know the sugar content, just keep fruit to a minimum (less than 2 pieces per day or 1 for a child). Juice or dried versions are not acceptable substitutes for whole fruit or vegetables.

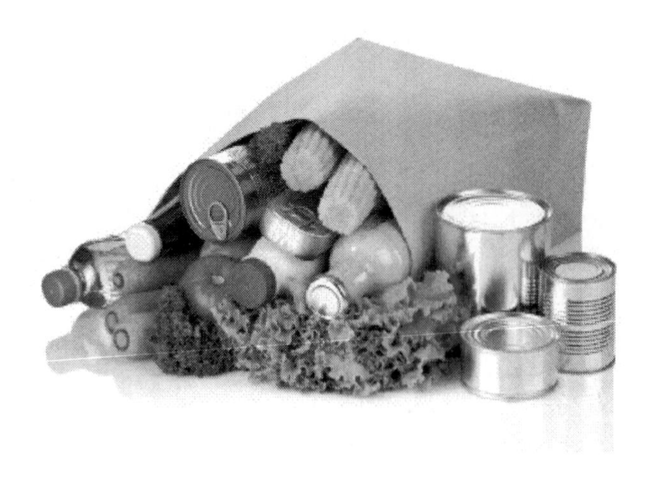

Sugar Substitutes

I'm not a big fan of the term artificial sweetener. It implies that other sweeteners (such as sugar, or fruit juice or high fructose corn syrup) are in some way natural, with all the goodness we have been conditioned to imply into that term. And there is nothing natural about extracting sugar from sugar cane. Substitute sweetener strikes me as a more appropriate description. They are substitutes for sugar, intended to do the job of sugar. In reality sugar itself is a substitute sweetener (for honey) but let's not get all technical. They are all created by using various levels of technology (from manmade beehives to industrial chemical plants) with the sole purpose of adding sweet taste to foods which are not otherwise sweet.

There are three categories of substitute sweetener; those that are absolutely safe to consume; and those that may be safe in limited doses and those which are not safe under any circumstances (usually because they are metabolized to fructose anyway).

Substitute Sweeteners commonly used in North America

Good	Your call	Bad	
Corn Syrup	Acesulphame potassium (#950)	Agave Syrup	Mannitol (#421)
Dextrose	Alitame (#956)	Fructose	Maple Syrup
Glucose	Aspartame (#951)	Fruit Juice Extract	Molasses
Glucose Syrup	Aspartame-acesuphame (#962)	Golden Syrup	Polydextrose
Lactose	Cyclamates (#952)	High Fructose Corn Syrup	Resistant (malto) dextrin
Maltose	Erythritol (#968)	Honey	Sorbitol (#420)
Maltodextrin	Neotame (#961)	Inulin	Sucrose
Maltodextrose	Saccharin (#954)	Isomalt (#953)	Wheat dextrin
Rice Malt Syrup	Stevia (#960)	Lactitol (#966)	
	Sucralose (#955)	Litesse	
	Xylitol (#967)	Maltitol (#965)	

Seed Oils

The lists that follow are based entirely on sugar content alone. I have also written about the dangers of some types of vegetable oil (seed oils) in my book Toxic Oil. Some of the products in the lists below will contain seed oils, but as food manufacturers are not required to label the exact fats that they are using in a product, I have not included information about the fats in these lists. We can however have an educated guess and if you are concerned about the seed oil content of any product, I encourage you to use my fat ready reckoner chart available at www.howmuchsugar.com.

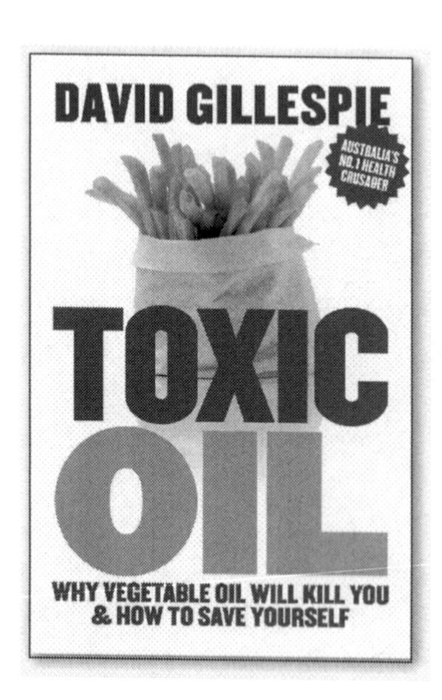

The Lists

Breakfast and Protein Bars 11

Drinks 13

Confectionery 14

Condiments

Condiments – by sugar content 15

Condiments – alphabetical 27

Salad Dressings 40

Cooking Sauces

Cooking Sauces – By Sugar Content 41

Cooking Sauces – alphabetical 49

Breakfast Cereals 59

Ice-Cream 61

Yogurts

Yogurts – by sugar content 64

Yogurts – alphabetical 72

Breads

Breads – by sugar content 80
Breads – alphabetical 84

Crackers

Crackers – by sugar content 88
Crackers – alphabetical 92

Frozen Pizza

Frozen Pizza – by sugar content 96
Frozen Pizza – alphabetical 103

Frozen Dinners

Frozen Dinners – by sugar content 110
Frozen Dinners – alphabetical 129

Boxed Meals

Boxed Meals – by sugar content 152
Boxed Meals – alphabetical 161

Fast Food

Subway Restaurants 171
McDonald's 175
Burger King 177
Pizza Hut 179
KFC 181
Taco Bell 183

Breakfast and Protein Bars

Label	% Sugar
Atkins Advantage Bar Triple Chocolate Bar	0.0%
Atkins Advantage Meal Bar Chocolate Chip Granola	0.0%
Pure Protein 78 Gram Protein Revolution	1.3%
Atkins Advantage Meal Bar Chocolate Peanut Butter	1.7%
Atkins Advantage Meal Bar Chocolate Chip Cookie Dough	1.7%
Quest Nutrition Protein Vanilla Almond Crunch	1.7%
Quest Nutrition Protein Chocolate Peanut Butter	1.7%
Quest Nutrition Protein Cinnamon Roll	1.7%
Quest Nutrition Protein Chocolate Brownie	1.7%
Quest Nutrition Protein Lemon Cream Pie	1.7%
Quest Nutrition Protein White Chocolate Raspberry	1.7%
Quest Nutrition Protein Double Chocolate Chunk	1.7%
Quest Nutrition Protein Choc Chip Cookie Dough	1.7%
Power Bar Protein & Recovery Chocolate Peanut Butter Reduced Sugar	1.7%
Quest Nutrition Cravings Peanut Butter Cups	2.0%
Pure Protein 50 Gram Protein Revolution	2.0%
Atkins Advantage Meal Bar Cinnamon Bun	2.1%
Atkins Advantage Meal Bar Cookies n' Crème	2.1%
Atkins Advantage Meal Bar Mudslide	2.1%
Atkins Advantage Meal Bar Peanut Butter Granola	2.1%
Atkins Advantage Meal Bar Peanut Fudge Granola	2.1%
Atkins Advantage Bar Caramel Chocolate Peanut Nougat	2.3%
Atkins Advantage Bar Caramel Double Chocolate Crunch	2.3%

Label	% Sugar
Atkins Advantage Bar Caramel Fudge Brownie	2.3%
Atkins Advantage Bar Coconut Almond Delight	2.3%
Atkins Advantage Bar Dark Chocolate Decadence	2.3%
Atkins Advantage Bar Dark Chocolate Almond Coconut Crunch	2.5%
Atkins Day Break Bar Chocolate Hazelnut	2.5%
Atkins Day Break Bar Chocolate Oatmeal Fiber	2.5%
Atkins Day Break Bar Oatmeal Cinnamon	2.5%
Atkins Day Break Bar Chocolate Chip Crisp	2.9%
Atkins Day Break Bar Cranberry Almond	2.9%
Atkins Day Break Bar Peanut Butter Fudge Crisp	2.9%

The Atkins Advantage, Pure Protein and Power Bar brands are very low in sugar but use artificial sweeteners which are metabolized to fructose (the ones on the 'Bad' list on previous page). The Quest Bars use sucralose or stevia (both on the 'Your Call' list).

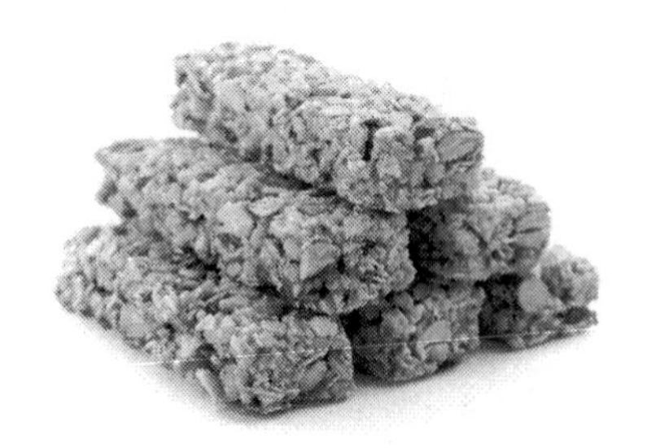

Drinks

The only qualifying products are unsweetened tea or coffee, diet soft drinks, water and milk (both whole and low fat).

Most diet versions of sodas are sweetened with a sweetener on the 'Your Call' list above.

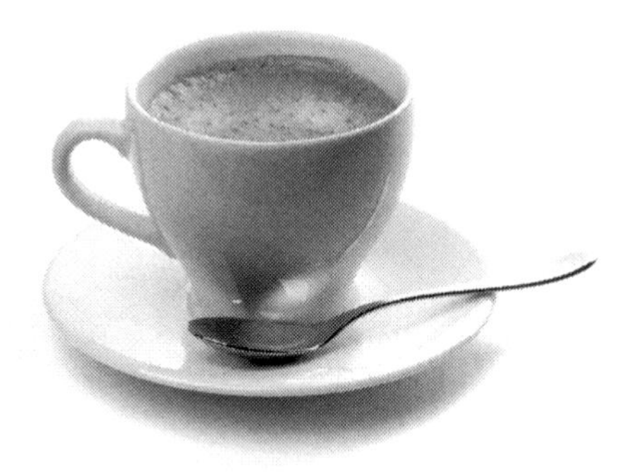

Confectionery

All of the following products have been sweetened with glucose rather than sugar (sucrose).

Maker	Product
Wonka (Nestle)	Runts
	Bottle Caps
	Everlasting Gobstopper
	Chewy Gobstopper
	Gobstopper Snowballs
Frusano	Filita Organic Whole Milk Chocolate
	Organic-Filita Amaranth
	Organic Rice-Crispies
	Filita Organic Dark Chocolate
	Organic Fili-Bears (Gummi Bears)
	Organic Blackberry Candies
	Organic Peppermint Candies
	Ricemalt peppermint hard candy
	Ricemalt lemon hard candy
	Ricemalt orange hard candy
	Dextrose Lolly

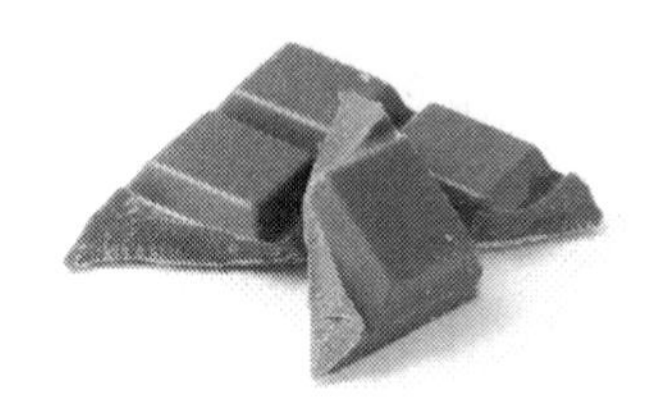

Condiments

Because there are so many choices in this category, I've presented this list in two formats so you can browse by sugar content or brand. Most of the low sugar versions of popular sauces use a sweetener on the 'your call' list above. If you prefer not to consume those you'll have to make them yourself. I have provided some easy-to-make recipes in The Sweet Poison Quit Plan. Most of these products contain seed oils so check the ingredient list on the labels carefully if you are being cautious of them.

Condiments - by sugar content

Product	% Sugar
Badia Mojo Marinade	0.0%
Beano's Buffalo Sandwich Sauce Deli Condiment	0.0%
Beano's Jalepeno Mustard Deli Condiment	0.0%
Beano's Smokey Bacon Sandwich Sauce Deli Condiment	0.0%
Best Foods Canola Cholesterol Free Mayonnaise	0.0%
Best Foods Southwestern Ranch Reduced Fat Mayonnaise	0.0%
Blue Plate Light Mayonnaise	0.0%
Blue Plate Light with Olive Oil Mayonnaise	0.0%
Blue Plate Real Mayonnaise	0.0%
Cholula Original Hot Sauce	0.0%
Cookies Wings-N-Things Hot Sauce	0.0%
Crosse & Blackwell Chow Chow	0.0%
Demler's Yellow Mustard	0.0%
Dickinson's Apricot Sugar Free Preserves	0.0%
Dickinson's Cherry Sugar Free Preserves	0.0%
Dickinson's Red Raspberry Sugar Free Preserves	0.0%

Condiments - by sugar content (continued)

Product	% Sugar
Dickinson's Seedless Blackberry Sugar Free Preserves	0.0%
Dickinson's Strawberry Sugar Free Preserves	0.0%
Duke's Cholesterol Free Mayonnaise	0.0%
Duke's Light Mayonnaise	0.0%
Duke's Light With Olive Oil Mayonnaise	0.0%
Duke's Original Mayonnaise	0.0%
Dulcet Moroccan Mustard	0.0%
El Diablo Jalapeno Hot & Spicy Mustard	0.0%
El Diablo Roasted Chipotle Hot & Spicy Mustard	0.0%
El Diablo Steakhouse Hot & Spicy Mustard	0.0%
El Pinto Medium Red Chile Sauce	0.0%
El Pinto Hot Enchilada Sauce	0.0%
El Pinto Medium Enchilada Sauce	0.0%
El Pinto Mild Enchilada Sauce	0.0%
El Yucateco Bisteck Paste	0.0%
El Yucateco Mayakut Sauce	0.0%
Emeril's Kicked Up Horseradish Mustard	0.0%
French's Dijon Mustard	0.0%
French's Horseradish Mustard	0.0%
Frontera Carne Asada Marinade	0.0%
Golding Farms Horseradish Mustard	0.0%
Grace Hot Pepper Sauce	0.0%
Great Value Loaded Baked Potato Dip	0.0%
Great Value Light Mayonnaise Mayonnaise	0.0%
Great Value Mayonnaise	0.0%
Great Value Coarse Ground Mustard	0.0%

Condiments - by sugar content (continued)

Product	% Sugar
Great Value Dijon Mustard	0.0%
Great Value Horseradish Mustard	0.0%
Great Value Spicy Brown Mustard	0.0%
Great Value Yellow Mustard	0.0%
Great Value Hot Dog Chili Sauce	0.0%
Great Value Sugar Free Blackberry Preserves	0.0%
Great Value Sugar Free Chocolate Syrup	0.0%
Grey Poupon Bistro Sauce Dijon Mustard	0.0%
Grey Poupon Classic Dijon Mustard	0.0%
Grey Poupon Country Dijon Mustard	0.0%
Gulden's Spicy Brown Mustard	0.0%
Gulden's Yellow Mustard	0.0%
Heinz Mayonnaise	0.0%
Heinz Yellow Mustard	0.0%
Hellmann's Canola Cholesterol Free Mayonnaise	0.0%
Hellmann's Light Mayonnaise	0.0%
Hellmann's Real Mayonnaise	0.0%
Hellmann's Southwestern Ranch Mayonnaise	0.0%
Herdez Queso Blanco Con Jalapenos Dip	0.0%
Hidden Valley Oven Roasted Garlic Parmesan Sandwich Spread	0.0%
Hidden Valley Smoked Bacon Sandwich Spread	0.0%
Hidden Valley Spicy Chipotle Pepper Sandwich Spread	0.0%
Huy Fong Chili Garlic Sauce	0.0%
Huy Fong Sambal Oelek Sauce	0.0%
Iberia Mayonnaise	0.0%

Condiments - by sugar content (continued)

Product	% Sugar
Jack Daniels Old No. 7 Mustard	0.0%
Jack Daniels Stone Ground Dijon Mustard	0.0%
Jardine's Campfire Roasted Salsa	0.0%
Jardine's Jalapeno Verde Salsa	0.0%
JFG Mayonnaise	0.0%
Ka-Me Hot Mustard	0.0%
Ken Davis Classic 2 Carb BBQ Sauce	0.0%
Kikkoman Wasabi Asian Sauce	0.0%
Kraft Mayo	0.0%
Kraft Sugar Free Cool Whip	0.0%
La Preferida Louisiana Hot Sauce	0.0%
La Preferida Taquera Salsa	0.0%
La Preferida Thick 'n Chunky Medium Salsa	0.0%
La Preferida Thick 'n Chunky Mild Salsa	0.0%
La Preferida Think 'n Chunky Hot Salsa	0.0%
La Preferida Mojo Marinade	0.0%
La Victoria Red Mild Enchilada Sauce	0.0%
La Victoria Chipotle Taco Sauce	0.0%
La Victoria Green Medium Taco Sauce	0.0%
La Victoria Green Mild Taco Sauce	0.0%
La Victoria Salsa Brava Taco Sauce	0.0%
Maranatha Creamy & Raw Sesame Tahiti	0.0%
Maranatha Roasted Sesame Tahiti	0.0%
Margaritaville Island Chipotle Dip	0.0%
Margaritaville Mild Island Garlic Guacamole	0.0%
Margaritaville Zesty Island Garlic Guacamole	0.0%

Condiments - by sugar content (continued)

Product	% Sugar
Margaritaville Chipotle Garlic Salsa	0.0%
Mezzetta Chimichurri Sandwich Spread	0.0%
Mission Cheddar Cheese Dip	0.0%
Naturally Fresh Buffalo Bleu Cheese Dip	0.0%
Old Dutch Nàcho Cheese Dip	0.0%
Old El Paso Medium Cheese & Salsa	0.0%
Old El Paso Mild Cheese & Salsa	0.0%
Old El Paso Medium Taco Sauce	0.0%
Organicville Dijon Mustard	0.0%
Organicville Stone Ground Mustard	0.0%
Organicville Yellow Mustard	0.0%
Ortega Green Taco Sauce	0.0%
Plochman's Mild Yellow Mustard	0.0%
Plochman's Stone Ground Mustard	0.0%
Polaner Orange Sugar Free Marmalade	0.0%
Polaner Apricot Sugar Free Preserves	0.0%
Price First Mayonnaise	0.0%
Price First Yellow Mustard	0.0%
Red Cactus Stadium Cheddar Cheese Sauce	0.0%
Salpica Cheddar Nacho Sauce	0.0%
Salpica Chipotle Black Bean Salsa	0.0%
Salpica Chipotle Garlic Salsa	0.0%
Salpica Cilantro Green Olive Salsa	0.0%
Salpica Jalapeno Jack Queso Salsa	0.0%
Salpica Roasted Corn & Bean Salsa	0.0%
Salpica Salsa Con Queso Salsa	0.0%

Condiments - by sugar content (continued)

Product	% Sugar
San J Organic Shoyu Soy Sauce	0.0%
San J Lite Tamari Soy Sauce	0.0%
San J Organic Tamari Soy Sauce	0.0%
San J Organic Reduced Sodium Tamari Soy Sauce	0.0%
San J Original Tamari Soy Sauce	0.0%
San J Reduced Sodium Tamari Soy Sauce	0.0%
Santa Barbara Hot Salsa	0.0%
Silver Spring Cream Style Horseradish	0.0%
Silver Spring Extra Hot Horseradish	0.0%
Silver Spring Fresh Ground Horseradish	0.0%
Silver Spring Organic Prepared Horseradish	0.0%
Silver Spring Prepared Horseradish	0.0%
Silver Spring With Beets Horseradish	0.0%
Silver Spring Beer 'n Brat Mustard	0.0%
Silver Spring Chipotle Mustard	0.0%
Silver Spring Deli Style Mustard	0.0%
Silver Spring Dijon Mustard	0.0%
Silver Spring Dill Mustard	0.0%
Silver Spring Habanero Mustard	0.0%
Silver Spring Jalapeno Mustard	0.0%
Silver Spring Mayo Blend Mustard	0.0%
Silver Spring Whole Grain Mustard	0.0%
Silver Spring Horseradish Sauce	0.0%
Silver Spring Mango Wasabi Sauce	0.0%
Smucker's Blackberry With Splenda Sugar Free Jam	0.0%
Smucker's Blackberry With Truvia Sugar Free Jam	0.0%

Condiments - by sugar content (continued)

Product	% Sugar
Smucker's Concord Grape Sugar Free Jam	0.0%
Smucker's Strawberry Sugar Free Jam	0.0%
Smucker's Orange Sugar Free Marmalade	0.0%
Smucker's Apricot Sugar Free Preserves	0.0%
Smucker's Blueberry Sugar Free Preserves	0.0%
Smucker's Boysenberry Sugar Free Preserves	0.0%
Smucker's Cherry Sugar Free Preserves	0.0%
Smucker's Peach Sugar Free Preserves	0.0%
Smucker's Red Raspberry Sugar Free Preserves	0.0%
Smucker's Strawberry With Splenda Sugar Free Preserves	0.0%
Smucker's Strawberry With Truvia Sugar Free Preserves	0.0%
Spectrum Canola Mayonnaise	0.0%
Spectrum Canola Light Mayonnaise	0.0%
Spectrum Olive Oil Mayonnaise	0.0%
Spectrum Omega 3 Mayonnaise	0.0%
Spectrum Organic Mayonnaise	0.0%
Sweet Baby Rays Creamy Buffalo Wing Dipping Sauce	0.0%
Taco Bell Fire Restaurant Sauce	0.0%
Taco Bell Hot Restaurant Sauce	0.0%
Taco Bell Mild Restaurant Sauce	0.0%
Tapatio Hot Sauce Hot Sauce	0.0%
Terrapin Ridge Farms Garam Masala Stoneground Mustard	0.0%
Terrapin Ridge Farms Smokey Onion Mustard	0.0%
Terrapin Ridge Farms Wasabi Lime Mustard	0.0%
Terrapin Ridge Farms Creamy Garlic Pretzel Dip	0.0%

Condiments - by sugar content (continued)

Product	% Sugar
Texas Pete Chipotle Hot Sauce	0.0%
Texas Pete Original Hot Sauce	0.0%
Texas Pete Fiery Sweet Wing Sauce	0.0%
The Ojai Cook Cha Cha Chipotle Lemonaise	0.0%
The Ojai Cook Fire & Spice Lemonaise	0.0%
The Ojai Cook Garlic Herb Lemonaise	0.0%
The Ojai Cook Green Dragon Lemonaise	0.0%
The Ojai Cook Latin Lemonaise	0.0%
The Ojai Cook Light Lemonaise	0.0%
The Ojai Cook Original Lemonaise	0.0%
The Ojai Cook Bite Back Tartar Sauce	0.0%
The Ojai Cook Smokey Chipotle Marinade	0.0%
Tostitos Smooth & Cheesy Dip	0.0%
Tostitos Zesty Taco Dip	0.0%
Tostitos Montery Jack Queso	0.0%
Try Me Yucatan Sunshine Habanero Sauce	0.0%
Ty Ling Hot Chinese Mustard	0.0%
Ty Ling Oyster Sauce	0.0%
Valentina Extra Hot Hot Sauce	0.0%
Valentina Original Hot Sauce	0.0%
Walden Farms Hickory Smoke BBQ Sauce	0.0%
Walden Farms Honey BBQ Sauce	0.0%
Walden Farms Original BBQ Sauce	0.0%
Walden Farms Thick 'N Spicy BBQ Sauce	0.0%
Walden Farms Bacon Dips	0.0%
Walden Farms Bleu Cheese Dips	0.0%

Condiments – by sugar content (continued)

Product	% Sugar
Walden Farms French Onion Dips	0.0%
Walden Farms Ranch Dips	0.0%
Walden Farms Ketchup	0.0%
Walden Farms Amazin' Mayo	0.0%
Walden Farms Chipotle Mayo	0.0%
Walden Farms Honey Mustard Mayo	0.0%
Walden Farms Pomegranate Mayo	0.0%
Walden Farms Ranch Mayo	0.0%
Walden Farms Apple Butter Fruit Spread	0.0%
Walden Farms Apricot Fruit Spread	0.0%
Walden Farms Cranberry Sauce Fruit Spread	0.0%
Walden Farms Grape Fruit Spread	0.0%
Walden Farms Raspberry Fruit Spread	0.0%
Walden Farms Strawberry Fruit Spread	0.0%
Walden Farms Caramel Dips	0.0%
Walden Farms Chocolate Dips	0.0%
Walden Farms Marshmallow Dips	0.0%
Walden Farms Caramel Syrup	0.0%
Walden Farms Chocolate Syrup	0.0%
Walden Farms Strawberry Syrup	0.0%
Westbrae Dijon Style Mustard	0.0%
Westbrae Stone Ground Mustard	0.0%
Westbrae Stone Ground No Salt Mustard	0.0%
Westbrae Yellow Mustard	0.0%
Woeber's Southwest Horseradish Sauce	0.0%
Woeber's Cool Dill Mayo Gourmet	0.0%

Condiments - by sugar content (continued)

Product	% Sugar
Woeber's Kickin' Buffalo Mayo Gourmet	0.0%
Woeber's Roasted Chipotle Mayo Gourmet	0.0%
Woeber's Smoky Bacon Mayo Gourmet	0.0%
Woeber's Toasted Garlic Mayo Gourmet	0.0%
Woeber's Dijon Mustard	0.0%
Woeber's Dusseldorf Mustard	0.0%
Woeber's Jalapeno Mustard	0.0%
Woeber's Salad Style Mustard	0.0%
Woeber's Spicy Brown Mustard	0.0%
Woeber's Deli Organic Mustard	0.0%
Woeber's Spicy Brown Organic Mustard	0.0%
Woeber's Yellow Organic Mustard	0.0%
Woeber's Champagne Dill Mustard Reserve	0.0%
Woeber's Whole Grain Dijon Mustard Reserve	0.0%
Woeber's Dijon Supreme Mustard	0.0%
Woeber's Wasabi Supreme Mustard	0.0%
Zatarain's Creole Mustard	0.0%
Zatarain's New Orleans Yellow Mustard	0.0%
Zatarain's Prepared Horseradish Prepared Horseradish	0.0%
El Rio Hot Nacho Cheese Sauce	1.6%
El Rio Mild Nacho Cheese Sauce	1.6%
El Rio Regular Nacho Cheese Sauce	1.6%
Old El Paso Mild Green Chile Enchilada Sauce	1.6%
Chi-Chi's Green Mild Enchilada Sauce	1.7%
Great Value Medium Enchilada Sauce	1.7%
Great Value Mild Enchilada Sauce	1.7%

Condiments - by sugar content (continued)

Product	% Sugar
Herdez Green Chili Enchilada Sauce	1.7%
Herdez Red Chili Enchilada Sauce	1.7%
La Victoria Green Mild Enchilada Sauce	1.7%
La Victoria Red Chile Enchilada Sauce	1.7%
La Victoria Red Hot Enchilada Sauce	1.7%
Old El Paso Hot Enchilada Sauce	1.7%
Old El Paso Medium Enchilada Sauce	1.7%
Old El Paso Mild Enchilada Sauce	1.7%
Ortega Mild Green Enchilada Sauce	1.7%
Ortega Mild Red Enchilada Sauce	1.7%
Texas Pete Seafood Cocktail Sauce	1.7%
Fischer & Wieser Black Bean & Corn Salsa	2.5%
Fischer & Wieser Hot Habanero Salsa	2.5%
Fischer & Wieser Salsa a La Charra Salsa	2.5%
Fischer & Wieser Salsa Verde Ranchera Salsa	2.5%
Mrs. Renfro's Ghost Pepper Salsa	2.6%
Mrs. Renfro's Habanero Salsa	2.6%
Ernie's Chesapeake Shrimp Salsa	2.9%
Texas Pete Extra Mild Buffalo Wing Sauce	2.9%
Tostitos Catalina Thick & Chunky Salsa	2.9%
World Table Spinach & Artichoke Dip	2.9%
Great Value Medium Con Queso Salsa	2.9%
Herdez Queso Con Salsa Dip	2.9%
Joe T. Garcia's Mild Salsa Picante	2.9%
Mission Salsa Con Queso Dip	2.9%
Old Dutch Salsa Con Queso Restaurant Style Dip	2.9%

Condiments - by sugar content (continued)

Product	% Sugar
On The Border Con Queso Salsa	2.9%
Texas Pete Buffalo Wing Sauce	2.9%
Tostitos Catalina Chipotle Salsa	2.9%
Tostitos Catalina Verde Salsa	2.9%
Mrs. Renfro's Black Bean Salsa	3.0%
Mrs. Renfro's Chipotle Corn Salsa	3.0%
Mrs. Renfro's Chipotle Nacho Cheese Sauce	3.0%
Mrs. Renfro's Ghost Pepper Nacho Cheese Sauce	3.0%
Mrs. Renfro's Nacho Cheese Sauce	3.0%

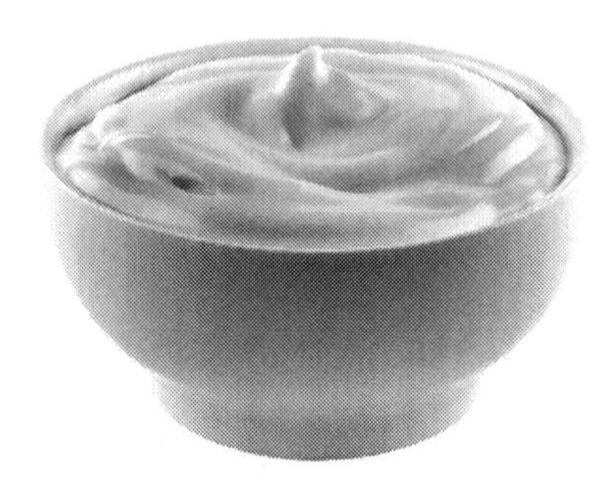

Condiments - alphabetical

Maker	Product	% Sugar
Badia	Badia Mojo Marinade	0.0%
Beano's	Beano's Buffalo Sandwich Sauce Deli Condiment	0.0%
	Beano's Jalepeno Mustard Deli Condiment	0.0%
	Beano's Smokey Bacon Sandwich Sauce Deli Condiment	0.0%
Best Foods	Best Foods Canola Cholesterol Free Mayonnaise	0.0%
	Best Foods Southwestern Ranch Reduced Fat Mayonnaise	0.0%
Blue Plate	Blue Plate Light Mayonnaise	0.0%
	Blue Plate Light with Olive Oil Mayonnaise	0.0%
Blue Plate	Blue Plate Real Mayonnaise	0.0%
Chi-Chi's	Chi-Chi's Green Mild Enchilada Sauce	1.7%
Cholula	Cholula Original Hot Sauce	0.0%
Cookies	Cookies Wings-N-Things Hot Sauce	0.0%
Crosse & Blackwell	Crosse & Blackwell Chow Chow	0.0%
Demler's	Demler's Yellow Mustard	0.0%
Dickinson's	Dickinson's Apricot Sugar Free Preserves	0.0%
	Dickinson's Cherry Sugar Free Preserves	0.0%
	Dickinson's Red Raspberry Sugar Free Preserves	0.0%
	Dickinson's Seedless Blackberry Sugar Free Preserves	0.0%
	Dickinson's Strawberry Sugar Free Preserves	0.0%

Condiments - alphabetical (continued)

Maker	Product	% Sugar
Duke's	Duke's Cholesterol Free Mayonnaise	0.0%
	Duke's Light Mayonnaise	0.0%
	Duke's Light With Olive Oil Mayonnaise	0.0%
	Duke's Original Mayonnaise	0.0%
Dulcet	Dulcet Moroccan Mustard	0.0%
El Diablo	El Diablo Jalapeno Hot & Spicy Mustard	0.0%
	El Diablo Roasted Chipotle Hot & Spicy Mustard	0.0%
	El Diablo Steakhouse Hot & Spicy Mustard	0.0%
El Pinto	El Pinto Medium Red Chile Sauce	0.0%
	El Pinto Hot Enchilada Sauce	0.0%
El Pinto	El Pinto Medium Enchilada Sauce	0.0%
	El Pinto Mild Enchilada Sauce	0.0%
El Rio	El Rio Hot Nacho Cheese Sauce	1.6%
	El Rio Mild Nacho Cheese Sauce	1.6%
	El Rio Regular Nacho Cheese Sauce	1.6%
El Yucateco	El Yucateco Bisteck Paste	0.0%
	El Yucateco Mayakut Sauce	0.0%
Emeril's	Emeril's Kicked Up Horseradish Mustard	0.0%
Ernie's	Ernie's Chesapeake Shrimp Salsa	2.9%
Fischer & Wieser	Fischer & Wieser Black Bean & Corn Salsa	2.5%
	Fischer & Wieser Hot Habanero Salsa	2.5%
	Fischer & Wieser Salsa a La Charra Salsa	2.5%
	Fischer & Wieser Salsa Verde Ranchera Salsa	2.5%

Condiments - alphabetical (continued)

Maker	Product	% Sugar
French's	French's Dijon Mustard	0.0%
	French's Horseradish Mustard	0.0%
Frontera	Frontera Carne Asada Marinade	0.0%
Golding Farms	Golding Farms Horseradish Mustard	0.0%
Grace	Grace Hot Pepper Sauce	0.0%
Great Value	Great Value Loaded Baked Potato Dip	0.0%
	Great Value Light Mayonnaise Mayonnaise	0.0%
	Great Value Mayonnaise	0.0%
	Great Value Coarse Ground Mustard	0.0%
	Great Value Dijon Mustard	0.0%
Great Value	Great Value Horseradish Mustard	0.0%
	Great Value Spicy Brown Mustard	0.0%
	Great Value Yellow Mustard	0.0%
	Great Value Hot Dog Chili Sauce	0.0%
	Great Value Sugar Free Blackberry Preserves	0.0%
	Great Value Sugar Free Chocolate Syrup	0.0%
	Great Value Medium Enchilada Sauce	1.7%
	Great Value Mild Enchilada Sauce	1.7%
	Great Value Medium Con Queso Salsa	2.9%
Grey Poupon	Grey Poupon Bistro Sauce Dijon Mustard	0.0%
	Grey Poupon Classic Dijon Mustard	0.0%
	Grey Poupon Country Dijon Mustard	0.0%
Gulden's	Gulden's Spicy Brown Mustard	0.0%
	Gulden's Yellow Mustard	0.0%

Condiments - alphabetical (continued)

Maker	Product	% Sugar
Heinz	Heinz Mayonnaise	0.0%
	Heinz Yellow Mustard	0.0%
Hellmann's	Hellmann's Canola Cholesterol Free Mayonnaise	0.0%
	Hellmann's Light Mayonnaise	0.0%
	Hellmann's Real Mayonnaise	0.0%
	Hellmann's Southwestern Ranch Mayonnaise	0.0%
Herdez	Herdez Queso Blanco Con Jalapenos Dip	0.0%
	Herdez Green Chili Enchilada Sauce	1.7%
	Herdez Red Chili Enchilada Sauce	1.7%
Herdez	Herdez Queso Con Salsa Dip	2.9%
Hidden Valley	Hidden Valley Oven Roasted Garlic Parmesan Sandwich Spread	0.0%
	Hidden Valley Smoked Bacon Sandwich Spread	0.0%
	Hidden Valley Spicy Chipotle Pepper Sandwich Spread	0.0%
Huy Fong	Huy Fong Chili Garlic Sauce	0.0%
	Huy Fong Sambal Oelek Sauce	0.0%
Iberia	Iberia Mayonnaise	0.0%
Jack Daniels	Jack Daniels Old No. 7 Mustard	0.0%
	Jack Daniels Stone Ground Dijon Mustard	0.0%
Jardine's	Jardine's Campfire Roasted Salsa	0.0%
	Jardine's Jalapeno Verde Salsa	0.0%
JFG	JFG Mayonnaise	0.0%

Condiments - alphabetical (continued)

Maker	Product	% Sugar
Joe T. Garcia's	Joe T. Garcia's Mild Salsa Picante	2.9%
Ka-Me	Ka-Me Hot Mustard	0.0%
Ken Davis	Ken Davis Classic 2 Carb BBQ Sauce	0.0%
Kikkoman	Kikkoman Wasabi Asian Sauce	0.0%
Kraft	Kraft Mayo	0.0%
	Kraft Sugar Free Cool Whip	0.0%
La Preferida	La Preferida Louisiana Hot Sauce	0.0%
	La Preferida Taquera Salsa	0.0%
	La Preferida Thick 'n Chunky Medium Salsa	0.0%
	La Preferida Thick 'n Chunky Mild Salsa	0.0%
La Preferida	La Preferida Think 'n Chunky Hot Salsa	0.0%
	La Preferida Mojo Marinade	0.0%
La Victoria	La Victoria Red Mild Enchilada Sauce	0.0%
	La Victoria Chipotle Taco Sauce	0.0%
	La Victoria Green Medium Taco Sauce	0.0%
	La Victoria Green Mild Taco Sauce	0.0%
	La Victoria Salsa Brava Taco Sauce	0.0%
	La Victoria Green Mild Enchilada Sauce	1.7%
	La Victoria Red Chile Enchilada Sauce	1.7%
	La Victoria Red Hot Enchilada Sauce	1.7%
Maranatha	Maranatha Creamy & Raw Sesame Tahiti	0.0%
	Maranatha Roasted Sesame Tahiti	0.0%
Margaritaville	Margaritaville Island Chipotle Dip	0.0%
	Margaritaville Mild Island Garlic Guacamole	0.0%

Condiments - alphabetical (continued)

Maker	Product	% Sugar
	Margaritaville Zesty Island Garlic Guacamole	0.0%
	Margaritaville Chipotle Garlic Salsa	0.0%
Mezzetta	Mezzetta Chimichurri Sandwich Spread	0.0%
Mission	Mission Cheddar Cheese Dip	0.0%
	Mission Salsa Con Queso Dip	2.9%
Mrs. Renfro's	Mrs. Renfro's Ghost Pepper Salsa	2.6%
	Mrs. Renfro's Habanero Salsa	2.6%
	Mrs. Renfro's Black Bean Salsa	3.0%
	Mrs. Renfro's Chipotle Corn Salsa	3.0%
Mrs. Renfro's	Mrs. Renfro's Chipotle Nacho Cheese Sauce	3.0%
	Mrs. Renfro's Ghost Pepper Nacho Cheese Sauce	3.0%
	Mrs. Renfro's Nacho Cheese Sauce	3.0%
Naturally Fresh	Naturally Fresh Buffalo Bleu Cheese Dip	0.0%
Old Dutch	Old Dutch Nacho Cheese Dip	0.0%
	Old Dutch Salsa Con Queso Restaurant Style Dip	2.9%
Old El Paso	Old El Paso Medium Cheese & Salsa	0.0%
	Old El Paso Mild Cheese & Salsa	0.0%
	Old El Paso Medium Taco Sauce	0.0%
	Old El Paso Mild Green Chile Enchilada Sauce	1.6%
	Old El Paso Hot Enchilada Sauce	1.7%
	Old El Paso Medium Enchilada Sauce	1.7%
	Old El Paso Mild Enchilada Sauce	1.7%

Condiments - alphabetical (continued)

Maker	Product	% Sugar
On The Border	On The Border Con Queso Salsa	2.9%
Organicville	Organicville Dijon Mustard	0.0%
	Organicville Stone Ground Mustard	0.0%
	Organicville Yellow Mustard	0.0%
Ortega	Ortega Green Taco Sauce	0.0%
	Ortega Mild Green Enchilada Sauce	1.7%
	Ortega Mild Red Enchilada Sauce	1.7%
Plochman's	Plochman's Mild Yellow Mustard	0.0%
	Plochman's Stone Ground Mustard	0.0%
Polaner	Polaner Orange Sugar Free Marmalade	0.0%
Polaner	Polaner Apricot Sugar Free Preserves	0.0%
Price First	Price First Mayonnaise	0.0%
	Price First Yellow Mustard	0.0%
Red Cactus	Red Cactus Stadium Cheddar Cheese Sauce	0.0%
Salpica	Salpica Cheddar Nacho Sauce	0.0%
	Salpica Chipotle Black Bean Salsa	0.0%
	Salpica Chipotle Garlic Salsa	0.0%
	Salpica Cilantro Green Olive Salsa	0.0%
	Salpica Jalapeno Jack Queso Salsa	0.0%
	Salpica Roasted Corn & Bean Salsa	0.0%
	Salpica Salsa Con Queso Salsa	0.0%
San J	San J Organic Shoyu Soy Sauce	0.0%
	San J Lite Tamari Soy Sauce	0.0%
	San J Organic Tamari Soy Sauce	0.0%
	San J Organic Reduced Sodium Tamari Soy Sauce	0.0%

Condiments - alphabetical (continued)

Maker	Product	% Sugar
	San J Original Tamari Soy Sauce	0.0%
	San J Reduced Sodium Tamari Soy Sauce	0.0%
Santa Barbara	Santa Barbara Hot Salsa	0.0%
Silver Spring	Silver Spring Cream Style Horseradish	0.0%
	Silver Spring Extra Hot Horseradish	0.0%
	Silver Spring Fresh Ground Horseradish	0.0%
	Silver Spring Organic Prepared Horseradish	0.0%
	Silver Spring Prepared Horseradish	0.0%
Silver Spring	Silver Spring With Beets Horseradish	0.0%
	Silver Spring Beer 'n Brat Mustard	0.0%
	Silver Spring Chipotle Mustard	0.0%
	Silver Spring Deli Style Mustard	0.0%
	Silver Spring Dijon Mustard	0.0%
	Silver Spring Dill Mustard	0.0%
	Silver Spring Habanero Mustard	0.0%
	Silver Spring Jalapeno Mustard	0.0%
	Silver Spring Mayo Blend Mustard	0.0%
	Silver Spring Whole Grain Mustard	0.0%
	Silver Spring Horseradish Sauce	0.0%
	Silver Spring Mango Wasabi Sauce	0.0%
Smucker's	Smucker's Blackberry With Splenda Sugar Free Jam	0.0%
	Smucker's Blackberry With Truvia Sugar Free Jam	0.0%
	Smucker's Concord Grape Sugar Free Jam	0.0%

Condiments - alphabetical (continued)

Maker	Product	% Sugar
	Smucker's Strawberry Sugar Free Jam	0.0%
	Smucker's Orange Sugar Free Marmalade	0.0%
	Smucker's Apricot Sugar Free Preserves	0.0%
	Smucker's Blueberry Sugar Free Preserves	0.0%
	Smucker's Boysenberry Sugar Free Preserves	0.0%
	Smucker's Cherry Sugar Free Preserves	0.0%
Smucker's	Smucker's Peach Sugar Free Preserves	0.0%
	Smucker's Red Raspberry Sugar Free Preserves	0.0%
	Smucker's Strawberry With Splenda Sugar Free Preserves	0.0%
	Smucker's Strawberry With Truvia Sugar Free Preserves	0.0%
Spectrum	Spectrum Canola Mayonnaise	0.0%
	Spectrum Canola Light Mayonnaise	0.0%
	Spectrum Olive Oil Mayonnaise	0.0%
	Spectrum Omega 3 Mayonnaise	0.0%
	Spectrum Organic Mayonnaise	0.0%
Sweet Baby Rays	Sweet Baby Rays Creamy Buffalo Wing Dipping Sauce	0.0%
Taco Bell	Taco Bell Fire Restaurant Sauce	0.0%
	Taco Bell Hot Restaurant Sauce	0.0%
	Taco Bell Mild Restaurant Sauce	0.0%
Tapatio	Tapatio Hot Sauce Hot Sauce	0.0%
Terrapin Ridge Farms	Terrapin Ridge Farms Garam Masala Stoneground Mustard	0.0%

Condiments - alphabetical (continued)

Maker	Product	% Sugar
	Terrapin Ridge Farms Smokey Onion Mustard	0.0%
	Terrapin Ridge Farms Wasabi Lime Mustard	0.0%
	Terrapin Ridge Farms Creamy Garlic Pretzel Dip	0.0%
Texas Pete	Texas Pete Chipotle Hot Sauce	0.0%
	Texas Pete Original Hot Sauce	0.0%
Texas Pete	Texas Pete Fiery Sweet Wing Sauce	0.0%
	Texas Pete Seafood Cocktail Sauce	1.7%
	Texas Pete Extra Mild Buffalo Wing Sauce	2.9%
	Texas Pete Buffalo Wing Sauce	2.9%
The Ojai Cook	The Ojai Cook Cha Cha Chipotle Lemonaise	0.0%
	The Ojai Cook Fire & Spice Lemonaise	0.0%
	The Ojai Cook Garlic Herb Lemonaise	0.0%
	The Ojai Cook Green Dragon Lemonaise	0.0%
	The Ojai Cook Latin Lemonaise	0.0%
	The Ojai Cook Light Lemonaise	0.0%
	The Ojai Cook Original Lemonaise	0.0%
	The Ojai Cook Bite Back Tartar Sauce	0.0%
	The Ojai Cook Smokey Chipotle Marinade	0.0%
Tostitos	Tostitos Smooth & Cheesy Dip	0.0%
	Tostitos Zesty Taco Dip	0.0%
	Tostitos Montery Jack Queso	0.0%
	Tostitos Catalina Thick & Chunky Salsa	2.9%

Condiments - alphabetical (continued)

Maker	Product	% Sugar
	Tostitos Catalina Chipotle Salsa	2.9%
	Tostitos Catalina Verde Salsa	2.9%
Try Me	Try Me Yucatan Sunshine Habanero Sauce	0.0%
Ty Ling	Ty Ling Hot Chinese Mustard	0.0%
	Ty Ling Oyster Sauce	0.0%
Valentina	Valentina Extra Hot Hot Sauce	0.0%
Valentina	Valentina Original Hot Sauce	0.0%
Walden Farms	Walden Farms Hickory Smoke BBQ Sauce	0.0%
	Walden Farms Honey BBQ Sauce	0.0%
	Walden Farms Original BBQ Sauce	0.0%
	Walden Farms Thick 'N Spicy BBQ Sauce	0.0%
	Walden Farms Bacon Dips	0.0%
	Walden Farms Bleu Cheese Dips	0.0%
	Walden Farms French Onion Dips	0.0%
	Walden Farms Ranch Dips	0.0%
	Walden Farms Ketchup	0.0%
	Walden Farms Amazin' Mayo	0.0%
	Walden Farms Chipotle Mayo	0.0%
	Walden Farms Honey Mustard Mayo	0.0%
	Walden Farms Pomegranate Mayo	0.0%
	Walden Farms Ranch Mayo	0.0%
	Walden Farms Apple Butter Fruit Spread	0.0%
	Walden Farms Apricot Fruit Spread	0.0%
	Walden Farms Cranberry Sauce Fruit Spread	0.0%

Condiments - alphabetical (continued)

Maker	Product	% Sugar
	Walden Farms Grape Fruit Spread	0.0%
	Walden Farms Raspberry Fruit Spread	0.0%
	Walden Farms Strawberry Fruit Spread	0.0%
	Walden Farms Caramel Dips	0.0%
	Walden Farms Chocolate Dips	0.0%
	Walden Farms Marshmallow Dips	0.0%
Walden Farms	Walden Farms Caramel Syrup	0.0%
	Walden Farms Chocolate Syrup	0.0%
	Walden Farms Strawberry Syrup	0.0%
Westbrae	Westbrae Dijon Style Mustard	0.0%
	Westbrae Stone Ground Mustard	0.0%
	Westbrae Stone Ground No Salt Mustard	0.0%
	Westbrae Yellow Mustard	0.0%
Woeber's	Woeber's Southwest Horseradish Sauce	0.0%
	Woeber's Cool Dill Mayo Gourmet	0.0%
	Woeber's Kickin' Buffalo Mayo Gourmet	0.0%
	Woeber's Roasted Chipotle Mayo Gourmet	0.0%
	Woeber's Smoky Bacon Mayo Gourmet	0.0%
	Woeber's Toasted Garlic Mayo Gourmet	0.0%
	Woeber's Dijon Mustard	0.0%
	Woeber's Dusseldorf Mustard	0.0%
	Woeber's Jalapeno Mustard	0.0%
	Woeber's Salad Style Mustard	0.0%
	Woeber's Spicy Brown Mustard	0.0%
	Woeber's Deli Organic Mustard	0.0%

Condiments - alphabetical (continued)

Maker	Product	% Sugar
	Woeber's Spicy Brown Organic Mustard	0.0%
	Woeber's Yellow Organic Mustard	0.0%
	Woeber's Champagne Dill Mustard Reserve	0.0%
	Woeber's Whole Grain Dijon Mustard Reserve	0.0%
Woeber's	Woeber's Dijon Supreme Mustard	0.0%
	Woeber's Wasabi Supreme Mustard	0.0%
World Table	World Table Spinach & Artichoke Dip	2.9%
Zatarain's	Zatarain's Creole Mustard	0.0%
	Zatarain's New Orleans Yellow Mustard	0.0%
	Zatarain's Prepared Horseradish Prepared Horseradish	0.0%

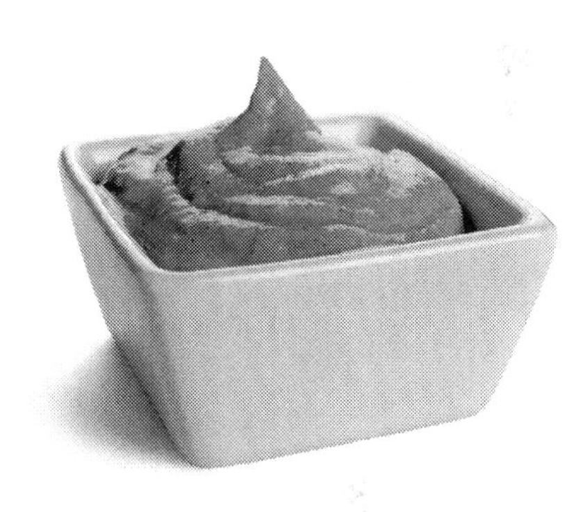

Salad Dressings

With dressings it seems you can have no sugar at all, or piles of the stuff. All of the following options are sugar free (all have 0 per cent sugar).

Salad Dressing
Bernstein's Cheese Fantastico
Bernstein's Creamy Caesar
Bernstein's Restaurant Recipe Italian
Cardini's Original Caesar
Gazebo Room Balsamic Vinaigrette
Gazebo Room Greek
Gazebo Room Lite Greek
Johnny's Great Caesar
Ken's Italian
Newman's Old Creamy Caesar
Newman's Old Family Recipe Italian
Newman's Old Lite Italian
Organicville Herbs De Provence
Organicville Sesame Tamari
Organicville Sun Dried Tomato & Garlic
Walden Farms Asian

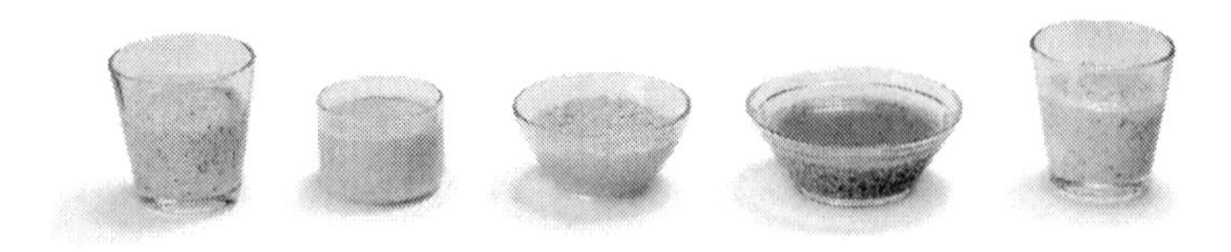

Cooking Sauces

These sauces are arranged by sugar content and then in a separate list by the maker. Be careful with the ones that say they are 0%. In many cases this is based on a very small serving size, and since in the US, labels are not required to state the amount per 100ml, it could be a misleading percentage. For this reason, I've also included the serving size this is based on.

Many of them contain also seed oils, so be careful if you are also aiming to avoid them.

Cooking Sauces - By Sugar Content

Serving size (g or ml)	Sugar per serve	Brand	% Sugar
5	0	Alessi Garlic Puree	0.0%
15	0	Badia Mojo Marinade	0.0%
125	0	Bar Harbor White Clam Sauce	0.0%
28	0	Beaver Tartar Sauce	0.0%
5	0	Cajun King Lemon Butter Amandine Sauce Mix	0.0%
2	0	Cajun King Barbecue Shrimp Sauce Mix	0.0%
60	0	Casa Fiesta Mild Enchilada Sauce	0.0%
15	0	China Bowl with Garlic Chilli Puree	0.0%
7	0	Concord Foods Potato Topping	0.0%
5	0	Dave's Hurtin Habenero Hot Sauce	0.0%
5	0	Dave's Insanity Hot Sauce	0.0%
5	0	Dave's Jalepeno Hot Sauce	0.0%
5	0	Dave's Total Insanity Hot Sauce	0.0%

Cooking Sauces - by sugar content (continued)

Serving size (g or ml)	Sugar per serve	Brand	% Sugar
35	0	Dell'Alpe Alla Genovese Pesto	0.0%
5	0	Dinosaur's Devil's Duel Hot Sauce	0.0%
28	0	Frisch's Original Tartar Sauce	0.0%
30	0	Gilway Mint Sauce	0.0%
5	0	Goya Hot Sauce	0.0%
5	0	Goya Cilantro Cooking Base	0.0%
60	0	Great Value Beef Gravy	0.0%
60	0	Great Value Chicken Gravy	0.0%
60	0	Great Value Turkey Gravy	0.0%
30	0	Guy Fieri Buffalo NY Wing Sauce	0.0%
19	0	Guy Fieri Hot Sugar Free BBQ Sauce	0.0%
19	0	Guy Fieri Original Sugar Free BBQ Sauce	0.0%
19	0	Guy Fieri Garlic Sugar Free BBQ Sauce	0.0%
19	0	Guy Fieri Spicy Sugar Free BBQ Sauce	0.0%
60	0	Hatch Fire-roasted Tomato Enchilada Sauce	0.0%
4.5	0	Herdez Jalepeno Hot Sauce	0.0%
28	0	Hooters 3 Mile Island Wing Sauce	0.0%
28	0	Hooters Hot Wing Sauce	0.0%
28	0	Hooters Medium Wing Sauce	0.0%
5	0	Jamaica Hell Fire Hot Sauce	0.0%
32	0	Jim Beam Wing Sauce	0.0%
20	0	Johnny's Au Jus French Dip	0.0%
123	0	La Costena Tomatillos	0.0%
5	0	La Preferida Enchilada Sauce	0.0%

Cooking Sauces - by sugar content (continued)

Serving size (g or ml)	Sugar per serve	Brand	% Sugar
5	0	La Preferida Traditional Louisiana Hot Sauce	0.0%
16	0	La Victoria Medium Green Taco Sauce	0.0%
16	0	La Victoria Mild Green Taco Sauce	0.0%
60	0	Las Palmas Green Chile Enchilada Sauce	0.0%
60	0	Las Palmas Hot Enchilada Sauce	0.0%
60	0	Las Palmas Medium Green Chile Enchilada Sauce	0.0%
60	0	Las Palmas Medium Red Chile Enchilada Sauce	0.0%
60	0	Las Palmas Mild Enchilada Sauce	0.0%
60	0	Las Palmas Red Chile Enchilada Sauce	0.0%
28.5	0	Louisiana Tartar Sauce	0.0%
15	0	McCormick Lemon Herb Seafood Sauce	0.0%
5	0	Mezzetta California Habenero Hot Sauce	0.0%
15	0	Mikey Brisket Cooking Sauce	0.0%
6	0	Mrs Wages Tomato Mix Pasta Sauce	0.0%
1.5	0	Orrington Farms Au Jus Mix Gravy	0.0%
60	0	Pacific Organic Turkey Gravy	0.0%
100	0	Patel's Lentil Curry	0.0%
63	0	Progresso Creamy Parmesan Basil Cooking Sauce	0.0%
63	0	Progresso Creamy Roasted Garlic Cooking Sauce	0.0%
15	0	Allegro Wild Game Game Tame Marinade	0.0%
15	0	Allegro Hot & Spicy Game Tame Marinade	0.0%

Cooking Sauces - by sugar content (continued)

Serving size (g or ml)	Sugar per serve	Brand	% Sugar
15	0	Allegro Soy & Lime Game Tame Marinade	0.0%
15	0	Cajun Injector Creole Garlic Injectable Marinade	0.0%
15	0	Cajun Injector Creole Butter Injectable Marinade	0.0%
15	0	Claude's Fajita Marinating Sauce	0.0%
4.5	0	Colgin Apple Liquid Smoke	0.0%
4.5	0	Colgin Original Liquid Smoke	0.0%
15	0	Drew's Buttermilk Ranch Dressing	0.0%
15	0	Drew's Italian Vinaigrette Dressing	0.0%
15	0	Drew's Rosemary Balsamic Dressing	0.0%
15	0	Drew's Soy Ginger Dressing	0.0%
15	0	Figaro Liquid Smoke Marinade	0.0%
30	0	Goya Jalepeno Hot Sauce	0.0%
30	0	Goya Mojo Marinade Marinade	0.0%
15	0	Great Value Less Sodium Soy Sauce	0.0%
15	0	House of Tsang Less Sodium Soy Sauce	0.0%
5	0	Ka-Me Fish Sauce	0.0%
12	0	Kikkoman Gluten Free Soy Sauce	0.0%
15	0	Kikkoman Less Sodium Soy Sauce	0.0%
15	0	Kikkoman Milder Soy Sauce	0.0%
15	0	Kikkoman Naturally brewed Soy Sauce	0.0%
15	0	Le Lechonera Mojo Criollo Marinade	0.0%
5	0	Louisiana Habenero Hot Sauce	0.0%
5	0	Louisiana Chipotle Hot Sauce	0.0%

Cooking Sauces - by sugar content (continued)

Serving size (g or ml)	Sugar per serve	Brand	% Sugar
5	0	Louisiana Roasted Garlic Hot Sauce	0.0%
5	0	LSU Hot Sauce	0.0%
5	0	Maggi Jugo Seasoning Sauce	0.0%
5	0	Melinda's Original Habenero Hot Sauce	0.0%
30	0	Milani Dill Sauce	0.0%
15	0	Moore's Buffalo Wing Sauce	0.0%
15	0	Moore's Buffalo Medium Wing Sauce	0.0%
15	0	Moore's Original Marinade	0.0%
61	1	El Rio with Jalepeno Cheese Sauce	0.0%
140	1	El Rio Hot Tamales Chilli Sauce	0.7%
129	1	Casa Visco Homestyle Spaghetti Sauce	0.8%
125	1	Alpino Hot & Spicy Pizza Sauce	0.8%
125	1	Dell'Alpe White Clam Sauce	0.8%
125	1	Marketside Creamy Alfredo Pasta Sauce	0.8%
124	1	Progresso White with Herb & Garlic Clam Sauce	0.8%
120	1	Cento White Clam Sauce	0.8%
113	1	Casa Corona Red Medium Enchilada Sauce	0.9%
113	1	Gia Russa Tomato Basil Pasta Sauce	0.9%
73	1	El Rio Mild Enchilada Sauce	1.4%
68	1	El Rio Hot Dog Chilli Sauce	1.5%
63	1	Progresso Creamy Portabella Mushroom Cooking Sauce	1.6%
62	1	Emeril's Roasted Garlic Alfredo Pasta Sauce	1.6%

Cooking Sauces - by sugar content (continued)

Serving size (g or ml)	Sugar per serve	Brand	% Sugar
123	2	Gia Russa Cherry Tomato Pasta Sauce	1.6%
61	1	Bertoli Alfredo Sauce	1.6%
61	1	Bertoli Garlic Alfredo Sauce	1.6%
61	1	Bertoli Mushroom Alfredo Sauce	1.6%
61	1	Bertoli Light Alfredo Sauce	1.6%
61	1	Contadina Roma Style Tomato Sauce	1.6%
61	1	Contadina Roma Style with Italian herbs Tomato Sauce	1.6%
61	1	El Rio Hot Nacho Cheese Sauce	1.6%
61	1	Francesco Rinaldi Alfredo Pasta Sauce	1.6%
61	1	Francesco Rinaldi Four Cheese Alfredo Pasta Sauce	1.6%
61	1	Newman's Own Roasted Garlic Alfredo Pasta Sauce	1.6%
61	1	Old El Paso Mild Green Chile Enchilada Sauce	1.6%
61	1	Ragu Classic Alfredo Pasta Sauce	1.6%
60	1	Classico Creamy Alfredo Light Pasta Sauce	1.7%
60	1	Classico Creamy Alfredo Pasta Sauce	1.7%
60	1	Classico Four Cheese Alfredo Pasta Sauce	1.7%
60	1	Classico Asiago Romano Alfredo Pasta Sauce	1.7%
60	1	Classico Roasted Garlic Alfredo Pasta Sauce	1.7%
60	1	Classico Roasted Poblano Alfredo Pasta Sauce	1.7%

Cooking Sauces - by sugar content (continued)

Serving size (g or ml)	Sugar per serve	Brand	% Sugar
60	1	Classico Roasted Red Pepper Alfredo Pasta Sauce	1.7%
60	1	Dawn Fresh Mushroom Steak Sauce	1.7%
60	1	Great Value Medium Enchilada Sauce	1.7%
60	1	Great Value Mild Enchilada Sauce	1.7%
60	1	Hatch Green Chile Enchilada Sauce	1.7%
60	1	Herdez Medium Red Chile Enchilada Sauce	1.7%
60	1	Herdez Mild Green Chile Enchilada Sauce	1.7%
60	1	Herdez Red Guajillo Chile Cooking Sauce	1.7%
60	1	Herdez Roasted Pasilla Chile Cooking Sauce	1.7%
60	1	Herdez Tomatillo Verde Cooking Sauce	1.7%
60	1	La Victoria Green Chile Mild Enchilada Sauce	1.7%
60	1	La Victoria Mild Traditional Enchilada Sauce	1.7%
60	1	La Victoria Hot Picante Enchilada Sauce	1.7%
60	1	Las Palmas Hot Green Chile Enchilada Sauce	1.7%
60	1	Old El Paso Hot Enchilada Sauce	1.7%
60	1	Old El Paso Mild Enchilada Sauce	1.7%
60	1	Campbell's Brown Gravy	1.7%
60	1	Campbell's Golden Pork Gravy	1.7%
60	1	Campbell's Beef Gravy	1.7%
60	1	Campbell's Creamy Parmesan Chicken Skillet Sauces	1.7%

Cooking Sauces - by sugar content (continued)

Serving size (g or ml)	Sugar per serve	Brand	% Sugar
60	1	Campbell's Moroccan Spice Slow Cooker Sauces	1.7%
113	2	Mareta with Beef Spaghetti Sauce	1.8%
64	1.5	Casa Visco Garlic Lover's California Style Pizza Sauce	2.3%
126	3	Del Monte Zesty Mild Green Chillies Diced Tomatoes	2.4%
126	3	Gia Russa Artichoke Pasta Sauce	2.4%
126	3	Gia Russa Puttanesca Pasta Sauce	2.4%
125	3	Bar Harbor Red Clam Sauce	2.4%
125	3	Bonavita Marinara Pasta Sauce	2.4%
125	3	Bonavita Tomato Basil Pasta Sauce	2.4%
125	3	Kitchens of India Mild Chili Pepper Curry	2.4%
125	3	Marketside Marinara Pasta Sauce	2.4%
123	3	Bonavita Vodka Pasta Sauce	2.4%
119	3	Bonavita Fra Diavolo Pasta Sauce	2.5%
119	3	Paesana Fra Diavolo Hot Sauce	2.5%
113	3	Gia Russa Alla Vodka Pasta Sauce	2.7%
113	3	Gia Russa Marinara Pasta Sauce	2.7%
35	1	Patak's Hot Curry Paste	2.9%
35	1	Patak's Madras Curry Paste	2.9%
35	1	Patak's Mild Curry Paste	2.9%
35	1	Patak's Tikka Marinade	2.9%
34	1	Dynasty Black Bean Garlic Sauce	2.9%

Cooking Sauces - alphabetical

Brand	Serving size (g or ml)	Sugar per serve	Label	% Sugar
Alessi	5	0	Alessi Garlic Puree	0.0%
Allegro	15	0	Allegro Wild Game Game Tame Marinade	0.0%
	15	0	Allegro Hot & Spicy Game Tame Marinade	0.0%
	15	0	Allegro Soy & Lime Game Tame Marinade	0.0%
Alpino	125	1	Alpino Hot & Spicy Pizza Sauce	0.8%
Badia	15	0	Badia Mojo Marinade	0.0%
Bar Harbor	125	0	Bar Harbor White Clam Sauce	0.0%
	125	3	Bar Harbor Red Clam Sauce	2.4%
Beaver	28	0	Beaver Tartar Sauce	0.0%
Bertoli	61	1	Bertoli Alfredo Sauce	1.6%
	61	1	Bertoli Garlic Alfredo Sauce	1.6%
	61	1	Bertoli Mushroom Alfredo Sauce	1.6%
	61	1	Bertoli Light Alfredo Sauce	1.6%
Bonavita	125	3	Bonavita Marinara Pasta Sauce	2.4%
	125	3	Bonavita Tomato Basil Pasta Sauce	2.4%
	123	3	Bonavita Vodka Pasta Sauce	2.4%
	119	3	Bonavita Fra Diavolo Pasta Sauce	2.5%
Cajun Injector	15	0	Cajun Injector Creole Garlic Injectable Marinade	0.0%

Cooking Sauces - alphabetical (continued)

Brand	Serving size (g or ml)	Sugar per serve	Label	% Sugar
Cajun Injector	15	0	Cajun Injector Creole Butter Injectable Marinade	0.0%
Cajun King	5	0	Cajun King Lemon Butter Amandine Sauce Mix	0.0%
	2	0	Cajun King Barbecue Shrimp Sauce Mix	0.0%
Campbell's	60	1	Campbell's Brown Gravy	1.7%
	60	1	Campbell's Golden Pork Gravy	1.7%
	60	1	Campbell's Beef Gravy	1.7%
	60	1	Campbell's Creamy Parmesan Chicken Skillet Sauces	1.7%
	60	1	Campbell's Moroccan Spice Slow Cooker Sauces	1.7%
Casa Corona	113	1	Casa Corona Red Medium Enchilada Sauce	0.9%
Casa Fiesta	60	0	Casa Fiesta Mild Enchilada Sauce	0.0%
Casa Visco	129	1	Casa Visco Homestyle Spaghetti Sauce	0.8%
	64	1.5	Casa Visco Garlic Lover's California Style Pizza Sauce	2.3%
Cento	120	1	Cento White Clam Sauce	0.8%
China Bowl	15	0	China Bowl with Garlic Chilli Puree	0.0%
Classico	60	1	Classico Creamy Alfredo Light Pasta Sauce	1.7%
	60	1	Classico Creamy Alfredo Pasta Sauce	1.7%

Cooking Sauces - alphabetical (continued)

Brand	Serving size (g or ml)	Sugar per serve	Label	% Sugar
Classico	60	1	Classico Four Cheese Alfredo Pasta Sauce	1.7%
	60	1	Classico Asiago Romano Alfredo Pasta Sauce	1.7%
	60	1	Classico Roasted Garlic Alfredo Pasta Sauce	1.7%
	60	1	Classico Roasted Poblano Alfredo Pasta Sauce	1.7%
	60	1	Classico Roasted Red Pepper Alfredo Pasta Sauce	1.7%
Claude's	15	0	Claude's Fajita Marinating Sauce	0.0%
Colgin	4.5	0	Colgin Apple Liquid Smoke	0.0%
	4.5	0	Colgin Original Liquid Smoke	0.0%
Concord Foods	7	0	Concord Foods Potato Topping	0.0%
Contadina	61	1	Contadina Roma Style Tomato Sauce	1.6%
	61	1	Contadina Roma Style with Italian herbs Tomato Sauce	1.6%
Dave's	5	0	Dave's Hurtin Habenero Hot Sauce	0.0%
	5	0	Dave's Insanity Hot Sauce	0.0%
	5	0	Dave's Jalepeno Hot Sauce	0.0%
	5	0	Dave's Total Insanity Hot Sauce	0.0%
Dawn Fresh	60	1	Dawn Fresh Mushroom Steak Sauce	1.7%

Cooking Sauces - alphabetical (continued)

Brand	Serving size (g or ml)	Sugar per serve	Label	% Sugar
Del Monte	126	3	Del Monte Zesty Mild Green Chillies Diced Tomatoes	2.4%
Dell'Alpe	35	0	Dell'Alpe Alla Genovese Pesto	0.0%
	125	1	Dell'Alpe White Clam Sauce	0.8%
Dinosaur's	5	0	Dinosaur's Devil's Duel Hot Sauce	0.0%
Drew's	15	0	Drew's Buttermilk Ranch Dressing	0.0%
	15	0	Drew's Italian Vinaigrette Dressing	0.0%
	15	0	Drew's Rosemary Balsamic Dressing	0.0%
	15	0	Drew's Soy Ginger Dressing	0.0%
Dynasty	34	1	Dynasty Black Bean Garlic Sauce	2.9%
El Rio	61	1	El Rio with Jalepeno Cheese Sauce	0.0%
	140	1	El Rio Hot Tamales Chilli Sauce	0.7%
	73	1	El Rio Mild Enchilada Sauce	1.4%
	68	1	El Rio Hot Dog Chilli Sauce	1.5%
	61	1	El Rio Hot Nacho Cheese Sauce	1.6%
Emeril's	62	1	Emeril's Roasted Garlic Alfredo Pasta Sauce	1.6%
Figaro	15	0	Figaro Liquid Smoke Marinade	0.0%

Cooking Sauces - alphabetical (continued)

Brand	Serving size (g or ml)	Sugar per serve	Label	% Sugar
Francesco Rinaldi	61	1	Francesco Rinaldi Alfredo Pasta Sauce	1.6%
	61	1	Francesco Rinaldi Four Cheese Alfredo Pasta Sauce	1.6%
Frisch's	28	0	Frisch's Original Tartar Sauce	0.0%
Gia Russa	113	1	Gia Russa Tomato Basil Pasta Sauce	0.9%
	123	2	Gia Russa Cherry Tomato Pasta Sauce	1.6%
	126	3	Gia Russa Artichoke Pasta Sauce	2.4%
	126	3	Gia Russa Puttanesca Pasta Sauce	2.4%
	113	3	Gia Russa Alla Vodka Pasta Sauce	2.7%
	113	3	Gia Russa Marinara Pasta Sauce	2.7%
Gilway	30	0	Gilway Mint Sauce	0.0%
Goya	5	0	Goya Hot Sauce	0.0%
	5	0	Goya Cilantro Cooking Base	0.0%
	30	0	Goya Jalepeno Hot Sauce	0.0%
	30	0	Goya Mojo Marinade Marinade	0.0%
Great Value	60	0	Great Value Beef Gravy	0.0%
	60	0	Great Value Chicken Gravy	0.0%
	60	0	Great Value Turkey Gravy	0.0%
	15	0	Great Value Less Sodium Soy Sauce	0.0%

Cooking Sauces - alphabetical (continued)

Brand	Serving size (g or ml)	Sugar per serve	Label	% Sugar
Great Value	60	1	Great Value Medium Enchilada Sauce	1.7%
	60	1	Great Value Mild Enchilada Sauce	1.7%
Guy Fieri	30	0	Guy Fieri Buffalo NY Wing Sauce	0.0%
	19	0	Guy Fieri Hot Sugar Free BBQ Sauce	0.0%
	19	0	Guy Fieri Original Sugar Free BBQ Sauce	0.0%
	19	0	Guy Fieri Garlic Sugar Free BBQ Sauce	0.0%
	19	0	Guy Fieri Spicy Sugar Free BBQ Sauce	0.0%
Hatch	60	0	Hatch Fire-roasted Tomato Enchilada Sauce	0.0%
	60	1	Hatch Green Chile Enchilada Sauce	1.7%
Herdez	4.5	0	Herdez Jalepeno Hot Sauce	0.0%
	60	1	Herdez Medium Red Chile Enchilada Sauce	1.7%
	60	1	Herdez Mild Green Chile Enchilada Sauce	1.7%
	60	1	Herdez Red Guajillo Chile Cooking Sauce	1.7%
	60	1	Herdez Roasted Pasilla Chile Cooking Sauce	1.7%
	60	1	Herdez Tomatillo Verde Cooking Sauce	1.7%

Cooking Sauces - alphabetical (continued)

Brand	Serving size (g or ml)	Sugar per serve	Label	% Sugar
Hooters	28	0	Hooters 3 Mile Island Wing Sauce	0.0%
	28	0	Hooters Hot Wing Sauce	0.0%
	28	0	Hooters Medium Wing Sauce	0.0%
House of Tsang	15	0	House of Tsang Less Sodium Soy Sauce	0.0%
Jamaica Hell Fire	5	0	Jamaica Hell Fire Hot Sauce	0.0%
Jim Beam	32	0	Jim Beam Wing Sauce	0.0%
Johnny's	20	0	Johnny's Au Jus French Dip	0.0%
Ka-Me	5	0	Ka-Me Fish Sauce	0.0%
Kikkoman	12	0	Kikkoman Gluten Free Soy Sauce	0.0%
	15	0	Kikkoman Less Sodium Soy Sauce	0.0%
	15	0	Kikkoman Milder Soy Sauce	0.0%
	15	0	Kikkoman Naturally brewed Soy Sauce	0.0%
Kitchens of India	125	3	Kitchens of India Mild Chili Pepper Curry	2.4%
La Costena	123	0	La Costena Tomatillos	0.0%
La Preferida	5	0	La Preferida Enchilada Sauce	0.0%
	5	0	La Preferida Traditional Louisiana Hot Sauce	0.0%
La Victoria	16	0	La Victoria Medium Green Taco Sauce	0.0%
	16	0	La Victoria Mild Green Taco Sauce	0.0%

Cooking Sauces - alphabetical (continued)

Brand	Serving size (g or ml)	Sugar per serve	Label	% Sugar
La Victoria	60	1	La Victoria Green Chile Mild Enchilada Sauce	1.7%
	60	1	La Victoria Mild Traditional Enchilada Sauce	1.7%
	60	1	La Victoria Hot Picante Enchilada Sauce	1.7%
Las Palmas	60	0	Las Palmas Green Chile Enchilada Sauce	0.0%
	60	0	Las Palmas Hot Enchilada Sauce	0.0%
	60	0	Las Palmas Medium Green Chile Enchilada Sauce	0.0%
	60	0	Las Palmas Medium Red Chile Enchilada Sauce	0.0%
	60	0	Las Palmas Mild Enchilada Sauce	0.0%
	60	0	Las Palmas Red Chile Enchilada Sauce	0.0%
	60	1	Las Palmas Hot Green Chile Enchilada Sauce	1.7%
Le Lechonera	15	0	Le Lechonera Mojo Criollo Marinade	0.0%
Louisiana	28.5	0	Louisiana Tartar Sauce	0.0%
	5	0	Louisiana Habenero Hot Sauce	0.0%
	5	0	Louisiana Chipotle Hot Sauce	0.0%
	5	0	Louisiana Roasted Garlic Hot Sauce	0.0%

Cooking Sauces - alphabetical (continued)

Brand	Serving size (g or ml)	Sugar per serve	Label	% Sugar
LSU	5	0	LSU Hot Sauce	0.0%
Maggi	5	0	Maggi Jugo Seasoning Sauce	0.0%
Mareta	113	2	Mareta with Beef Spaghetti Sauce	1.8%
Marketside	125	1	Marketside Creamy Alfredo Pasta Sauce	0.8%
	125	3	Marketside Marinara Pasta Sauce	2.4%
McCormick	15	0	McCormick Lemon Herb Seafood Sauce	0.0%
Melinda's	5	0	Melinda's Original Habenero Hot Sauce	0.0%
Mezzetta	5	0	Mezzetta California Habenero Hot Sauce	0.0%
Mikey	15	0	Mikey Brisket Cooking Sauce	0.0%
Milani	30	0	Milani Dill Sauce	0.0%
Moore's	15	0	Moore's Buffalo Wing Sauce	0.0%
	15	0	Moore's Buffalo Medium Wing Sauce	0.0%
	15	0	Moore's Original Marinade	0.0%
Mrs Wages	6	0	Mrs Wages Tomato Mix Pasta Sauce	0.0%
Newman's Own	61	1	Newman's Own Roasted Garlic Alfredo Pasta Sauce	1.6%
Old El Paso	61	1	Old El Paso Mild Green Chile Enchilada Sauce	1.6%

Cooking Sauces - alphabetical (continued)

Brand	Serving size (g or ml)	Sugar per serve	Label	% Sugar
Old El Paso	60	1	Old El Paso Hot Enchilada Sauce	1.7%
	60	1	Old El Paso Mild Enchilada Sauce	1.7%
Orrington Farms	1.5	0	Orrington Farms Au Jus Mix Gravy	0.0%
Pacific Organic	60	0	Pacific Organic Turkey Gravy	0.0%
Paesana	119	3	Paesana Fra Diavolo Hot Sauce	2.5%
Patak's	35	1	Patak's Hot Curry Paste	2.9%
	35	1	Patak's Madras Curry Paste	2.9%
	35	1	Patak's Mild Curry Paste	2.9%
	35	1	Patak's Tikka Marinade	2.9%
Patel's	100	0	Patel's Lentil Curry	0.0%
Progresso	63	0	Progresso Creamy Parmesan Basil Cooking Sauce	0.0%
	63	0	Progresso Creamy Roasted Garlic Cooking Sauce	0.0%
	124	1	Progresso White with Herb & Garlic Clam Sauce	0.8%
	63	1	Progresso Creamy Portabella Mushroom Cooking Sauce	1.6%
Ragu	61	1	Ragu Classic Alfredo Pasta Sauce	1.6%

Breakfast Cereals

Brand	Label	% Sugar
Better Oats	Oat Revolution Classic	0.0%
Fiber One	Fiber One	0.0%
Kashi	7 Whole Grain Puffs	0.0%
Malt-O-Meal	Hot Wheat Creamy	0.0%
Malt-O-Meal	Hot Wheat Original	0.0%
Mom's Best Naturals	Old Fashioned Oats	0.0%
Mom's Best Naturals	Quick Oats	0.0%
Mom's Best Naturals	Toasted Wheat-Fuls	0.0%
Nature's Path	Corn Puffs	0.0%
Nature's Path	Kamut Puffs	0.0%
Nature's Path	Millet Puffs	0.0%
Nature's Path	Rice Puffs	0.0%
Post	Shredded Wheat Original	0.0%
Quaker	Instant Grits Butter	0.0%
Quaker	Instant Grits Country Bacon	0.0%
Quaker	Instant Grits Original	0.0%
Quaker	Instant Oatmeal Original	0.0%
Quaker	Organic Instant Oatmeal Regular	0.0%
Quaker	Puffed Rice	0.0%
Quaker	Puffed Wheat	0.0%
Quaker	Quick Grits	0.0%
Kellogg's	Mini-Wheat Unfrosted	1.7%
Quaker	Weight Control Instant Oatmeal Banana Bread	2.2%

Brand	Label	% Sugar
Quaker	Weight Control Instant Oatmeal Cinnamon	2.2%
Quaker	Weight Control Instant Oatmeal Maple & Brown Sugar	2.2%
Quaker	Oats Old Fashioned	2.5%
Quaker	Oats Quick Oats	2.5%
Quaker	Oats Steel Cut	2.5%

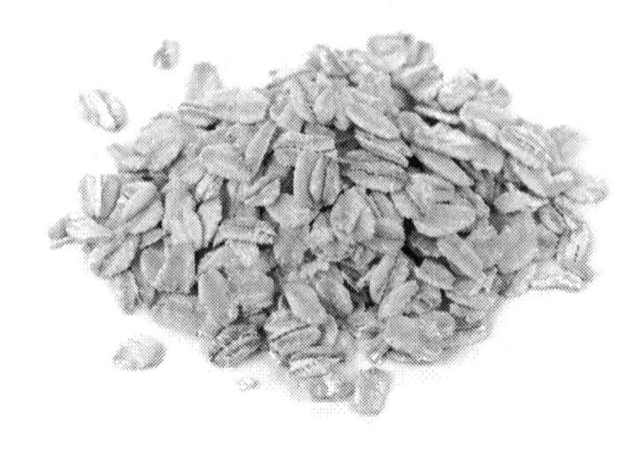

Ice-Cream

You'll see that I've used a column called 'Adjusted Sugar'. This is a calculated amount based on removing the 4.7 grams of lactose that the typical yogurt contains. Lactose is a galactose molecule joined to a glucose molecule. The galactose molecule is metabolised to glucose by your liver and lactose is therefore essentially pure glucose and fructose free. Lactose does not count towards your 3g per 100g limit.

Label	Adjusted Sugar	Artificial Sweetener
Dreyer's/Edy's No Sugar Added Slowchurned Ice Cream Butter Pecan	0%	1,2,3,4
Dreyer's/Edy's No Sugar Added Slowchurned Ice Cream Fudge Tracks	0%	1,2,3,4
Dreyer's/Edy's No Sugar Added Slowchurned Ice Cream Mint Chocolate Chip	0%	1,2,3,4
Dreyer's/Edy's No Sugar Added Slowchurned Ice Cream Triple Chocolate	0%	1,2,3,4
Blue Bunny Sweet Freedom Ice Cream Bars Krunch Lites	0%	1,3
Blue Bunny Sweet Freedom Ice Cream Bars Black Raspberry	1%	1,3
Dreyer's/Edy's No Sugar Added Slowchurned Ice Cream Vanilla Chocolate Swirl	1%	1,2,3,4
Blue Bunny Sweet Freedom Ice Cream Bars Fudge Lites	1%	1,3
Breyers Carb Smart Chocolate	1%	2,3,4,5
Breyers Carb Smart Vanilla	1%	2,3,4,5
Fudgsicle Ice Cream Bars No Sugar Added Fudge	1%	4,5,6,7
Dreyer's/Edy's No Sugar Added Slowchurned Ice Cream French Vanilla	2%	1,2,3,4

Label	Adjusted Sugar	Artificial Sweetener
Dreyer's/Edy's No Sugar Added Slowchurned Ice Cream Neopolitan	2%	1,2,3,4
Dreyer's/Edy's No Sugar Added Slowchurned Ice Cream Vanilla	2%	1,2,3,4
Dreyer's/Edy's No Sugar Added S lowchurned Ice Cream Vanilla Bean	2%	1,2,3,4
Breyers No Sugar Added Ice Cream Vanilla	2%	2,3,4
Breyers No Sugar Added Ice Cream Vanilla-Chocolate-Strawberry	2%	2,3,4
Blue Bunny Sweet Freedom No Sugar Added Ice Cream Banana Split	2%	2,4
Blue Bunny Sweet Freedom No Sugar Added Ice Cream Bunny Tracks	2%	2,4
Blue Bunny Sweet Freedom No Sugar Added Ice Cream Caramel Toffee Crunch	2%	2,4
Blue Bunny Sweet Freedom No Sugar Added Ice Cream Turtle Sundae	2%	2,4
Blue Bunny Sweet Freedom No Sugar Added Ice Cream Chocolate	3%	2,4
Blue Bunny Sweet Freedom No Sugar Added Ice Cream Vanilla	3%	2,4
Blue Bunny Sweet Freedom No Sugar Added Ice Cream Mint Chocolate Chip	3%	2,4
Blue Bell No Sugar Added Ice Cream Country Vanilla	3%	2,4,6

Key to the Sweeteners used

1. Maltitol (Bad)
2. Sorbitol (Bad)
3. Sucralose (Your Call)
4. Acesulphame potassium (Your Call)
5. Polydextrose (Bad)
6. Aspartame (Your Call)
7. Lactitol (Bad)

You won't be surprised to find that there no store bought ice-creams which satisfy the rule (without using a dubious sweetener). Even a small bowl (8 oz) of the lowest-sugar (not sweetened artificially) ice-cream (Ben & Jerry's Everything but the...) delivers two and a half teaspoons of added sugar. You'll be pleased to discover that I do provide a great recipe for sugar-free ice-cream in the recipe sections of howmuchsugar.com, in the Quit Plan Cookbook and in the Sweet Poison Quit Plan. Unfortunately, however, you have to make it yourself; no manufacturer yet makes ice-cream this way.)

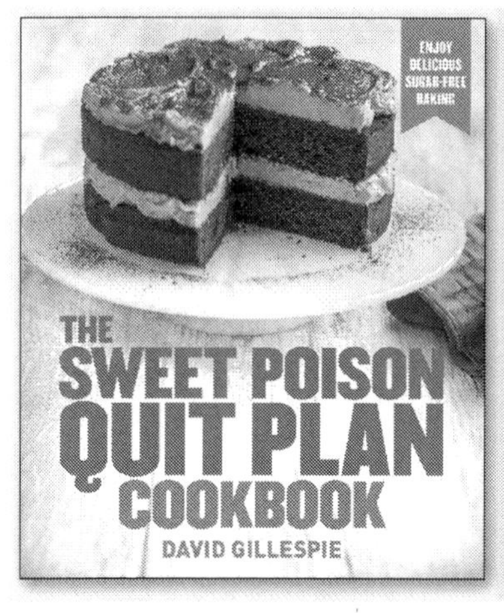

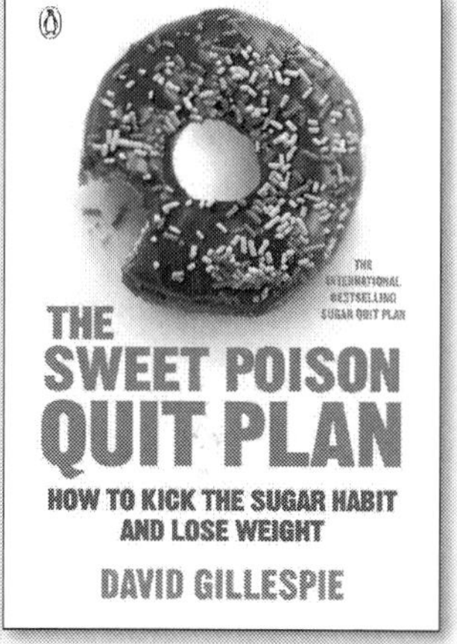

Yogurts

I've presented this list in two formats so you can browse by sugar content or brand. You'll see that I've used a column called 'Adjusted Sugar'. This is a calculated amount based on removing the 4.7 grams of lactose that the typical yogurt contains. Lactose is a galactose molecule joined to a glucose molecule. The galactose molecule is metabolised to glucose by your liver and lactose is therefore essentially pure glucose and fructose free. Lactose does not count towards your 3g per 100g limit.

Yogurts - by sugar content

Product	Adjusted Sugar
Dannon Strawberries & Cream Light & Fit Carb & Sugar Control	0.0%
Dannon Vanilla Cream Light & Fit Carb & Sugar Control	0.0%
Chobani Non-Fat Plain Blended	0.0%
Chobani Low-Fat Plain Blended	0.0%
Liberté Plain Greek	0.0%
Upstate Farms Plain Greek Yogurt	0.0%
Dannon French Onion Oikos Greek Yogurt Dips	0.0%
Dannon Cucumber Dill Oikos Greek Yogurt Dips	0.0%
Dannon Vegetable and Herb Oikos Greek Yogurt Dips	0.0%
Great Value Plain Greek Yogurt	0.0%
Dannon Plain Oikos Greek Nonfat Yogurt	0.0%
Dannon Plain Oikos Traditional Greek Yogurt	0.0%
Dannon Strawberry Light & Fit Greek	0.0%
Dannon Plain Light & Fit Greek	0.0%
Stoneyfield Plain Greek	0.0%

Yogurts - by sugar content (continued)

Product	Adjusted Sugar
Fage Plain Total Classic	0.0%
Fage Plain Total 2%	0.0%
Chobani Black Cherry Simply 100	0.0%
Chobani Pineapple Simply 100	0.0%
Chobani Peach Simply 100	0.0%
Belfonte Plain Greek Yogurt	0.0%
Fage Plain Toal 0%	0.0%
Lala Plain Yogurt	0.0%
Dannon Mixed Berry Light DanActive	0.0%
Dannon Strawberry Light DanActive	0.0%
Dannon Banana Cream Light & Fit Greek	0.0%
Dannon Blackberry Light & Fit Greek	0.0%
Dannon Blueberry Light & Fit Greek	0.0%
Dannon Caramel Macchiato Light & Fit Greek	0.0%
Dannon Key Lime Light & Fit Greek	0.0%
Dannon Peach Light & Fit Greek	0.0%
Dannon Pineapple Light & Fit Greek	0.0%
Dannon Pomegranate Berry Light & Fit Greek	0.0%
Dannon Raspberry Light & Fit Greek	0.0%
Dannon Strawberry Banana Light & Fit Greek	0.0%
Dannon Strawberry Cheesecake Light & Fit Greek	0.0%
Dannon Toasted Coconut Vanilla Light & Fit Greek	0.0%
Dannon Vanilla Light & Fit Greek	0.0%
Yoplait Key Lime Greek 100	0.0%
Yoplait Vanilla Greek 100	0.0%

Yogurts - by sugar content (continued)

Product	Adjusted Sugar
Chobani Strawberry Simply 100	0.0%
Chobani Vanilla Simply 100	0.0%
El Mexicano Vanilla Blended Yogurt	0.0%
Belfonte Blackberry & Crème Nonfat Yogurt	0.0%
Dannon Plain All Natural	0.6%
Stoneyfield Plain Whole Milk Smooth & Creamy	0.6%
Dannon Blueberry Light & Fit	0.6%
Dannon Strawberry Banana Light & Fit	0.6%
Brown Cow Plain Cream Top	0.6%
Hiland Dairy Vanilla Fat Free Yogurt	0.6%
Hiland Dairy Strawberry Fat Free Yogurt	0.6%
Hiland Dairy Peach Fat Free Yogurt	0.6%
Hiland Dairy Blueberry Fat Free Yogurt	0.6%
Belfonte Birthday Cake Nonfat Yogurt	0.6%
Belfonte Black Cherry Nonfat Yogurt	0.6%
Belfonte Cinnamon Roll Nonfat Yogurt	0.6%
Belfonte Red Velvet Cake Nonfat Yogurt	0.6%
Dannon Key Lime Activia Light	0.6%
Dannon Vanilla Activia Light	0.6%
Stoneyfield Plain YoBaby	0.6%
Mountain High Plain Original	0.6%
Dannon Cherry Light & Fit Greek	0.6%
Yoplait Apple Pie Greek 100	0.6%
Yoplait Strawberry Cheesecake Greek 100	0.6%
Chobani Blueberry Simply 100	0.6%

Yogurts - by sugar content (continued)

Product	Adjusted Sugar
La Yogurt Whole Milk Plain Family Style	1.0%
Brown Cow Plain Cream Top Greek	1.0%
Mountain High Plain Low Fat	1.1%
Dannon Banana Light & Fit	1.2%
Dannon Cherry Light & Fit	1.2%
Dannon Cherry Vanilla Light & Fit	1.2%
Dannon Key Lime Light & Fit	1.2%
Dannon Peach Light & Fit	1.2%
Dannon Pineapple Coconut Light & Fit	1.2%
Dannon Strawberry Cheesecake Light & Fit	1.2%
Dannon Vanilla Light & Fit	1.2%
Dannon Raspberry Goji Light & Fit	1.2%
Dannon Blueberry Acai Light & Fit	1.2%
Dannon Toasted Coconut Vanilla Light & Fit	1.2%
Yoplait Apple Turnover Light	1.2%
Yoplait Apricot Mango Light	1.2%
Yoplait Banana Cream Pie Light	1.2%
Yoplait Black Forrest Cake Light	1.2%
Yoplait Blackberry Light	1.2%
Yoplait Blueberry Patch Light	1.2%
Yoplait Boston Cream Pie Light	1.2%
Yoplait Harvest Peach Light	1.2%
Yoplait Key Lime Pie Light	1.2%
Yoplait Lemon Cream Pie Light	1.2%
Yoplait Orange Crème Light	1.2%

Yogurts - by sugar content (continued)

Product	Adjusted Sugar
Yoplait Pineapple Upside Down Cake Light	1.2%
Yoplait Raspberry Cheesecake Light	1.2%
Yoplait Raspberry Lemonade Light	1.2%
Yoplait Red Raspberry Light	1.2%
Yoplait Red Velvet Cake Light	1.2%
Yoplait Strawberries n Bananas Light	1.2%
Yoplait Strawberry Light	1.2%
Yoplait Strawberry Orange Sunrise Light	1.2%
Yoplait Strawberry Shortcake Light	1.2%
Yoplait Triple Berry Torte Light	1.2%
Yoplait Vanilla Cherry Light	1.2%
Yoplait Very Cherry Light	1.2%
Yoplait Very Vanilla Light	1.2%
Yoplait White Chocolate Strawberry Light	1.2%
Hiland Dairy Strawberry Banana Fat Free Yogurt	1.2%
Hiland Dairy Raspberry Fat Free Yogurt	1.2%
Hiland Dairy Cherry Vanilla Fat Free Yogurt	1.2%
Hiland Dairy Black Cherry Fat Free Yogurt	1.2%
Belfonte Apple Cobbler Nonfat Yogurt	1.2%
Belfonte Banana Crème Pie Nonfat Yogurt	1.2%
Belfonte Boston Cream Pie Nonfat Yogurt	1.2%
Belfonte Cherry Vanilla Nonfat Yogurt	1.2%
Belfonte Peach Nonfat Yogurt	1.2%
Belfonte Pomegrante Blueberry Nonfat Yogurt	1.2%
Belfonte Pomegranate Cherry Nonfat Yogurt	1.2%

Yogurts – by sugar content (continued)

Product	Adjusted Sugar
Belfonte Red Raspberry Nonfat Yogurt	1.2%
Belfonte Strawberry Nonfat Yogurt	1.2%
Belfonte Strawberry Banana Nonfat Yogurt	1.2%
Belfonte Orange Tango Nonfat Yogurt	1.2%
Yoplait Black Cherry Greek 100	1.3%
Yoplait Lemon Greek 100	1.3%
Yoplait Mixed Berry Greek 100	1.3%
Yoplait Peach Greek 100	1.3%
Yoplait Strawberry Greek 100	1.3%
Yoplait Tropical Greek 100	1.3%
Darigold Plain Yogurt	1.5%
Dannon Strawberry Banana Activia Light	1.5%
Dannon Strawberry Activia Light	1.5%
Dannon Raspberry Activia Light	1.5%
Dannon Peach Activia Light	1.5%
Dannon Blueberry Activia Light	1.5%
Mountain High Plain Fat Free	1.5%
Upstate Farms Plain Nonfat Yogurt	1.5%
Dannon Roasted Red Pepper Oikos Greek Yogurt Dips	1.6%
Dannon Pomegranate Berry Light & Fit	1.8%
Dannon Raspberry Light & Fit	1.8%
Dannon Strawberry Light & Fit	1.8%
Stoneyfield Plain Low Fat Smooth & Creamy	1.8%
La Yogurt Banana Cream Light	1.8%
La Yogurt Lemo Raspberry Light	1.8%

Yogurts - by sugar content (continued)

Product	Adjusted Sugar
La Yogurt Vanilla Light	1.8%
Great Value Strawberry Nonfat Yogurt	1.8%
Great Value Strawberry Banana Nonfat Yogurt	1.8%
Great Value Blueberry Nonfat Yogurt	1.8%
Belfonte Blueberry Nonfat Yogurt	1.8%
Belfonte Vanilla Nonfat Yogurt	1.8%
Crowley Strawberry Banana Burst Nonfat Yogurt	1.8%
La Yogurt Lowfat Plain Family Style	1.9%
Brown Cow Plain Low Fat	1.9%
Brown Cow Plain Nonfat	1.9%
La Yogurt Nonfat Plain Family Style	2.3%
Dannon Low Fat All Natural	2.4%
Dannon Non Fat All Natural	2.4%
Stoneyfield Plain Fat Free Smooth & Creamy	2.4%
La Yogurt Apple Pie Light	2.4%
La Yogurt Blueberry Light	2.4%
La Yogurt Coconut Pineapple Light	2.4%
La Yogurt Peach Light	2.4%
La Yogurt Pomegranate Berry Medley Light	2.4%
La Yogurt Raspberry Light	2.4%
La Yogurt Strawberry Light	2.4%
La Yogurt Strawberry Banana Light	2.4%
Great Value Orange Crème Pie Nonfat Yogurt	2.4%
Great Value Banana Cream Pie Nonfat Yogurt	2.4%
Great Value Vanilla Nonfat Yogurt	2.4%

Yogurts - by sugar content (continued)

Product	Adjusted Sugar
Great Value Peach Nonfat Yogurt	2.4%
Great Value Cherry Nonfat Yogurt	2.4%
Great Value Key Lime Pie Nonfat Yogurt	2.4%
Great Value Raspberry Nonfat Yogurt	2.4%
Belfonte White Chocolate Cherry Nonfat Yogurt	2.4%
Crowley Lovin' Lemon Nonfat Yogurt	2.4%
Crowley Bask In Banana Cream Nonfat Yogurt	2.4%
Crowley Peach Paradise Nonfat Yogurt	2.4%
Great Value Pina Colada Nonfat Yogurt	2.4%
La Yogurt Cherry Light	2.9%
Hiland Dairy Pomegranate Mango Fat Free Yogurt	2.9%
Hiland Dairy Lemon Fat Free Yogurt	2.9%
Hiland Dairy Apple and Spice Fat Free Yogurt	2.9%
Belfonte Coconut Cream Pie Nonfat Yogurt	2.9%
Belfonte Honey Almond Cream Nonfat Yogurt	2.9%
Belfonte Key Lime Pie Nonfat Yogurt	2.9%
Belfonte Strawberry Cheesecake Nonfat Yogurt	2.9%

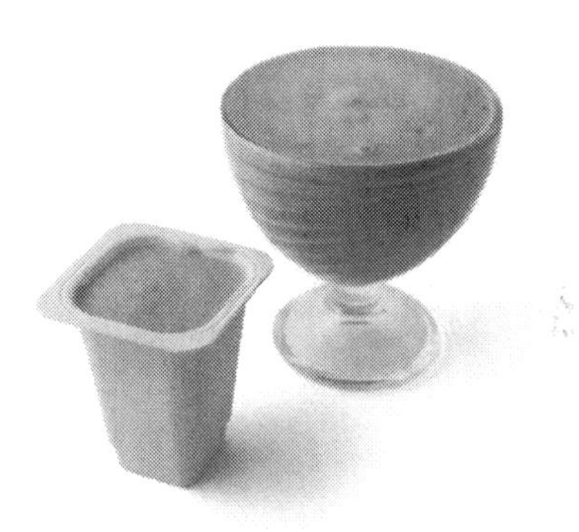

Yogurts - alphabetical

Maker	Product	Sub Product	Adjusted Sugar
Belfonte	Greek Yogurt	Plain	0.0%
	Nonfat Yogurt	Blackberry & Crème	0.0%
	Nonfat Yogurt	Birthday Cake	0.6%
	Nonfat Yogurt	Black Cherry	0.6%
	Nonfat Yogurt	Cinnamon Roll	0.6%
	Nonfat Yogurt	Red Velvet Cake	0.6%
	Nonfat Yogurt	Apple Cobbler	1.2%
	Nonfat Yogurt	Banana Crème Pie	1.2%
	Nonfat Yogurt	Boston Cream Pie	1.2%
	Nonfat Yogurt	Cherry Vanilla	1.2%
	Nonfat Yogurt	Peach	1.2%
	Nonfat Yogurt	Pomegrante Blueberry	1.2%
	Nonfat Yogurt	Pomegranate Cherry	1.2%
	Nonfat Yogurt	Red Raspberry	1.2%
	Nonfat Yogurt	Strawberry	1.2%
	Nonfat Yogurt	Strawberry Banana	1.2%
	Nonfat Yogurt	Orange Tango	1.2%
	Nonfat Yogurt	Blueberry	1.8%
	Nonfat Yogurt	Vanilla	1.8%
	Nonfat Yogurt	White Chocolate Cherry	2.4%
	Nonfat Yogurt	Coconut Cream Pie	2.9%
	Nonfat Yogurt	Honey Almond Cream	2.9%
	Nonfat Yogurt	Key Lime Pie	2.9%
	Nonfat Yogurt	Strawberry Cheesecake	2.9%
Brown Cow	Cream Top	Plain	0.6%

Yogurts - alphabetical (continued)

Maker	Product	Sub Product	Adjusted Sugar
Brown Cow	Cream Top Greek	Plain	1.0%
	Low Fat	Plain	1.9%
	Nonfat	Plain	1.9%
Chobani	Simply 100	Strawberry	0.0%
	Simply 100	Vanilla	0.0%
	Blended	Non-Fat Plain	0.0%
	Blended	Low-Fat Plain	0.0%
	Simply 100	Black Cherry	0.0%
	Simply 100	Pineapple	0.0%
	Simply 100	Peach	0.0%
	Simply 100	Blueberry	0.6%
Crowley	Nonfat Yogurt	Strawberry Banana Burst	1.8%
	Nonfat Yogurt	Lovin' Lemon	2.4%
	Nonfat Yogurt	Bask In Banana Cream	2.4%
	Nonfat Yogurt	Peach Paradise	2.4%
Dannon	Light & Fit Greek	Banana Cream	0.0%
	Light & Fit Greek	Blackberry	0.0%
	Light & Fit Greek	Blueberry	0.0%
	Light & Fit Greek	Caramel Macchiato	0.0%
	Light & Fit Greek	Key Lime	0.0%
	Light & Fit Greek	Peach	0.0%
	Light & Fit Greek	Pineapple	0.0%
	Light & Fit Greek	Pomegranate Berry	0.0%
	Light & Fit Greek	Raspberry	0.0%

Yogurts - alphabetical (continued)

Maker	Product	Sub Product	Adjusted Sugar
Dannon	Light & Fit Greek	Strawberry Banana	0.0%
	Light & Fit Greek	Strawberry Cheesecake	0.0%
	Light & Fit Greek	Toasted Coconut Vanilla	0.0%
	Light & Fit Greek	Vanilla	0.0%
	Light & Fit Carb & Sugar Control	Strawberries & Cream	0.0%
	Light & Fit Carb & Sugar Control	Vanilla Cream	0.0%
	Oikos Greek Yogurt Dips	French Onion	0.0%
	Oikos Greek Yogurt Dips	Cucumber Dill	0.0%
	Oikos Greek Yogurt Dips	Vegetable and Herb	0.0%
	Oikos Greek Nonfat Yogurt	Plain	0.0%
	Oikos Traditional Greek Yogurt	Plain	0.0%
	Light & Fit Greek	Strawberry	0.0%
	Light & Fit Greek	Plain	0.0%
	DanActive	Mixed Berry Light	0.0%
	DanActive	Strawberry Light	0.0%
	All Natural	Plain	0.6%
	Light & Fit	Blueberry	0.6%
	Light & Fit	Strawberry Banana	0.6%
	Activia Light	Key Lime	0.6%
	Activia Light	Vanilla	0.6%
	Light & Fit Greek	Cherry	0.6%

Yogurts - alphabetical (continued)

Maker	Product	Sub Product	Adjusted Sugar
Dannon	Light & Fit	Banana	1.2%
	Light & Fit	Cherry	1.2%
	Light & Fit	Cherry Vanilla	1.2%
	Light & Fit	Key Lime	1.2%
	Light & Fit	Peach	1.2%
	Light & Fit	Pineapple Coconut	1.2%
	Light & Fit	Strawberry Cheesecake	1.2%
	Light & Fit	Vanilla	1.2%
	Light & Fit	Raspberry Goji	1.2%
	Light & Fit	Blueberry Acai	1.2%
	Light & Fit	Toasted Coconut Vanilla	1.2%
	Activia Light	Strawberry Banana	1.5%
	Activia Light	Strawberry	1.5%
	Activia Light	Raspberry	1.5%
	Activia Light	Peach	1.5%
	Activia Light	Blueberry	1.5%
	Oikos Greek Yogurt Dips	Roasted Red Pepper	1.6%
	Light & Fit	Pomegranate Berry	1.8%
	Light & Fit	Raspberry	1.8%
	Light & Fit	Strawberry	1.8%
	All Natural	Low Fat	2.4%
	All Natural	Non Fat	2.4%
Darigold	Yogurt	Plain	1.5%
El Mexicano	Blended Yogurt	Vanilla	0.0%

Yogurts - alphabetical (continued)

Maker	Product	Sub Product	Adjusted Sugar
Fage	Total Classic	Plain	0.0%
	Total 2%	Plain	0.0%
Fage	Total 0%	Plain	0.0%
Great Value	Greek Yogurt	Plain	0.0%
	Nonfat Yogurt	Strawberry	1.8%
	Nonfat Yogurt	Strawberry Banana	1.8%
	Nonfat Yogurt	Blueberry	1.8%
	Nonfat Yogurt	Orange Crème Pie	2.4%
	Nonfat Yogurt	Banana Cream Pie	2.4%
	Nonfat Yogurt	Vanilla	2.4%
	Nonfat Yogurt	Peach	2.4%
	Nonfat Yogurt	Cherry	2.4%
	Nonfat Yogurt	Key Lime Pie	2.4%
	Nonfat Yogurt	Raspberry	2.4%
	Nonfat Yogurt	Pina Colada	2.4%
Hiland Dairy	Fat Free Yogurt	Vanilla	0.6%
	Fat Free Yogurt	Strawberry	0.6%
	Fat Free Yogurt	Peach	0.6%
	Fat Free Yogurt	Blueberry	0.6%
	Fat Free Yogurt	Strawberry Banana	1.2%
	Fat Free Yogurt	Raspberry	1.2%
	Fat Free Yogurt	Cherry Vanilla	1.2%
	Fat Free Yogurt	Black Cherry	1.2%
	Fat Free Yogurt	Pomegranate Mango	2.9%

Yogurts - alphabetical (continued)

Maker	Product	Sub Product	Adjusted Sugar
Hiland Dairy	Fat Free Yogurt	Lemon	2.9%
	Fat Free Yogurt	Apple and Spice	2.9%
La Yogurt	Family Style	Whole Milk Plain	1.0%
	Light	Banana Cream	1.8%
La Yogurt	Light	Lemo Raspberry	1.8%
	Light	Vanilla	1.8%
	Family Style	Lowfat Plain	1.9%
	Family Style	Nonfat Plain	2.3%
	Light	Apple Pie	2.4%
	Light	Blueberry	2.4%
	Light	Coconut Pineapple	2.4%
	Light	Peach	2.4%
	Light	Pomegranate Berry Medley	2.4%
	Light	Raspberry	2.4%
	Light	Strawberry	2.4%
	Light	Strawberry Banana	2.4%
	Light	Cherry	2.9%
Lala	Yogurt	Plain	0.0%
Liberté	Greek	Plain	0.0%
Mountain High	Original	Plain	0.6%
	Low Fat	Plain	1.1%
	Fat Free	Plain	1.5%
Stoneyfield	Greek	Plain	0.0%
	Smooth & Creamy	Plain Whole Milk	0.6%

Yogurts - alphabetical (continued)

Maker	Product	Sub Product	Adjusted Sugar
Stoneyfield	YoBaby	Plain	0.6%
	Smooth & Creamy	Plain Low Fat	1.8%
	Smooth & Creamy	Plain Fat Free	2.4%
Upstate Farms	Greek Yogurt	Plain	0.0%
	Nonfat Yogurt	Plain	1.5%
Yoplait	Greek 100	Key Lime	0.0%
	Greek 100	Vanilla	0.0%
	Greek 100	Apple Pie	0.6%
	Greek 100	Strawberry Cheesecake	0.6%
	Light	Apple Turnover	1.2%
	Light	Apricot Mango	1.2%
	Light	Banana Cream Pie	1.2%
	Light	Black Forrest Cake	1.2%
	Light	Blackberry	1.2%
	Light	Blueberry Patch	1.2%
	Light	Boston Cream Pie	1.2%
	Light	Harvest Peach	1.2%
	Light	Key Lime Pie	1.2%
	Light	Lemon Cream Pie	1.2%
	Light	Orange Crème	1.2%
	Light	Pineapple Upside Down Cake	1.2%
	Light	Raspberry Cheesecake	1.2%
	Light	Raspberry Lemonade	1.2%
	Light	Red Raspberry	1.2%

Yogurts – alphabetical (continued)

Maker	Product	Sub Product	Adjusted Sugar
Yoplait	Light	Red Velvet Cake	1.2%
	Light	Strawberries n Bananas	1.2%
	Light	Strawberry	1.2%
	Light	Strawberry Orange Sunrise	1.2%
	Light	Strawberry Shortcake	1.2%
	Light	Triple Berry Torte	1.2%
	Light	Vanilla Cherry	1.2%
	Light	Very Cherry	1.2%
	Light	Very Vanilla	1.2%
	Light	White Chocolate Strawberry	1.2%
	Greek 100	Black Cherry	1.3%
	Greek 100	Lemon	1.3%
	Greek 100	Mixed Berry	1.3%
	Greek 100	Peach	1.3%
	Greek 100	Strawberry	1.3%
	Greek 100	Tropical	1.3%

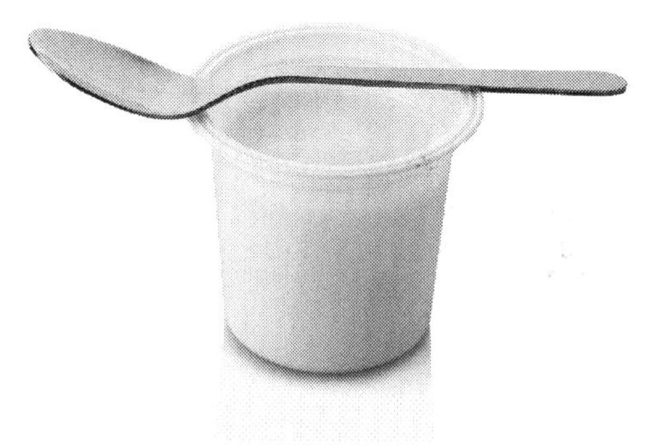

Breads

I've presented this list in two formats so you can browse by sugar content or brand. Almost all of the supermarket brands of bread contain rapeseed oil or another seed oil. If you are concerned about seed oil content then you will need to read the labels carefully. ***Avoid any that say they contain 'Vegetable Oil'***

Breads - by sugar content

Maker	Product	Percent Sugar
Feldkamp	Whole Rye Bread	0.0%
Feldkamp	Sunflower Seed Bread	0.0%
Ener-G	Brown Rice Yeast-Free Loaf	0.0%
Old London	Sourdough Melba Toast	0.0%
Feldkamp	Three Grain Bread	0.0%
Mestemacher	Sunflower Seed Bread	0.0%
Old London	Ancient Grains Melba Toast	0.0%
Mestemacher	Whole Rye Bread	0.0%
Ener-G	White Rice Yeast-Free Loaf	0.0%
Old London	Rye Melba Toast	0.0%
Old London	Wheat Melba Toast	0.0%
Old London	No Salt Whole Grain Melba Toast	0.0%
Old London	Whole Grain Melba Toast	0.0%
Old London	Classic Melba Toast	0.0%
Old London	Rosemary & Olive Oil Melba Toast	0.0%
Old London	Sesame Melba Toast	0.0%
Alvarado St. Bakery	Tortillas	0.0%
Taliano	Sliced Italian Bread	0.0%

Breads - by sugar content (continued)

Maker	Product	Percent Sugar
Nature's Own	100% Whole Wheat Whole Grain Bread	0.0%
Nature's Own	Whole Grain Sugar Free Bread	0.0%
Freihofer	Premium Italian Sourdough	0.0%
Freihofer	Brown 'N Serve Dinner Rolls	0.0%
Seattle International	Vienna Sourdough Bread	0.0%
Seattle International	French Baguette	0.0%
Seattle International	Classic Sourdough Bread	0.0%
Seattle Sourdough Baking Co.	Old Town Sourdough Bread	0.0%
Seattle Sourdough Baking Co.	Parmesan Garlic Sourdough Bread	0.0%
Mrs. Baird's	Sugar Free Whole Grain Wheat Bread	0.0%
The Bakery	Seeded Rye Bread	0.8%
The Bakery	Pumpernickel Bread	0.8%
Freihofer	Family White Bread	1.0%
Nature's Own	40 Calorie White Bread	1.1%
Great Value	White Enriched Bread	1.2%
Francisco	Sourdough Bread	1.2%
Arnold	Country Sourdough Bread	1.2%
Mestemacher	Fitness Bread	1.4%
Feldkamp	Pumpernickel Bread	1.5%
Pepperidge Farm	Jewish Rye Seedless Bread	1.6%
Pepperidge Farm	Deli Swirl Rye & Pump Bread	1.6%
Arnold	Premium Italian	1.6%
Freihofer	Italiano Seeded Bread	1.6%

Breads - by sugar content (continued)

Maker	Product	Percent Sugar
Freihofer	Italiano Unseeded Bread	1.6%
Freihofer	Premium Italian Bread	1.6%
Freihofer	Premium Italian Seeded Bread	1.6%
Freihofer	Sourdough Italiano!	1.6%
Franz	Extra Crisp English Muffins	1.6%
Franz	Plain English Muffins	1.6%
Franz	Sourdough English Muffins	1.6%
Freihofer	Soft Rye No Seeds	1.7%
Freihofer	Soft Rye Seeded	1.7%
Marketside	Pumpernickel Loaf Bread	1.8%
Marketside	Seeded Rye Loaf Bread	1.8%
Nature's Own	Double Fiber Wheat Bread	1.8%
Seattle Sourdough Baking Co.	Waterfront Sourdough Bread	1.8%
Nature's Own	100% Whole Wheat Bread	1.9%
Franz	Deli Sourdough	2.0%
Alvarado St. Bakery	Sprouted Wheat Bagel	2.1%
Aunt Millie's	Healthy Goodness Light Potato Bread	2.1%
Aunt Millie's	Healthy Goodness Light Whole Grain Bread	2.1%
Alvarado St. Bakery	Essential Flax Seed Bread	2.2%
Sara Lee	Delightful White Bread	2.2%
Natural Valley	Light Italian Sourdough Bread	2.2%
Nature's Own	Sourdough Bread	2.2%
Nature's Own	40 Calorie Wheat Bread	2.2%
Freihofer	Bulkie Rolls	2.4%

Breads - by sugar content (continued)

Maker	Product	Percent Sugar
Freihofer	Bulkie Rolls With Seeds	2.4%
Aunt Millie's	Hearth Whole Grain Deli Rye	2.5%
Holsum	Deli Rye Bread	2.5%
Holsum	Deli Sourdough	2.5%
Alvarado St. Bakery	Sprouted Whole Wheat Bread	2.6%
Aunt Millie's	German Rye Bread	2.6%
Freihofer	Country White Bread	2.8%
Franz	Deli Sourdough French Bread	2.8%
Alvarado St. Bakery	Sprouted Soy Crunch Bread	2.9%
Alvarado St. Bakery	California Style Bread	2.9%
Aunt Millie's	Homestyle 100% Whole Wheat Bread	2.9%
Aunt Millie's	Family Style Seeded Italian Bread	2.9%
Wheat Montana Farms	6 Carb, Wheat & Fibre Bread	2.9%
Franz	Italian Sandwich Bread	2.9%

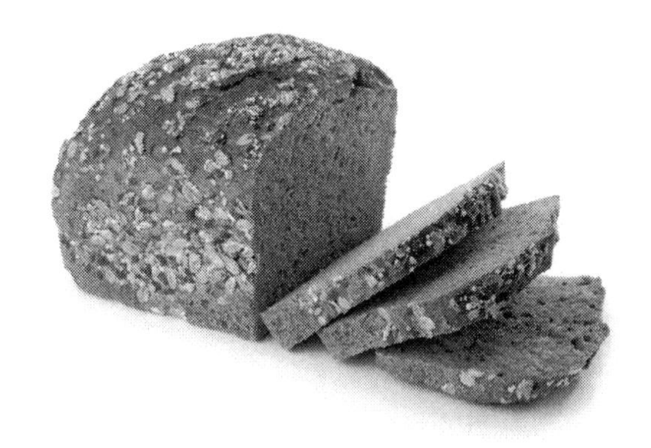

Breads - alphabetical

Maker	Product	Percent Sugar
Alvarado St. Bakery	Tortillas	0.0%
	Sprouted Wheat Bagel	2.1%
	Essential Flax Seed Bread	2.2%
	Sprouted Whole Wheat Bread	2.6%
	Sprouted Soy Crunch Bread	2.9%
	California Style Bread	2.9%
Arnold	Country Sourdough Bread	1.2%
	Premium Italian	1.6%
Aunt Millie's	Healthy Goodness Light Potato Bread	2.1%
	Healthy Goodness Light Whole Grain Bread	2.1%
	Hearth Whole Grain Deli Rye	2.5%
	German Rye Bread	2.6%
	Homestyle 100% Whole Wheat Bread	2.9%
	Family Style Seeded Italian Bread	2.9%
Ener-G	Brown Rice Yeast-Free Loaf	0.0%
	White Rice Yeast-Free Loaf	0.0%
Feldkamp	Whole Rye Bread	0.0%
	Sunflower Seed Bread	0.0%
	Three Grain Bread	0.0%
	Pumpernickel Bread	1.5%
Francisco	Sourdough Bread	1.2%
Franz	Extra Crisp English Muffins	1.6%
	Plain English Muffins	1.6%

Breads - alphabetical (continued)

Maker	Product	Percent Sugar
Franz	Sourdough English Muffins	1.6%
	Deli Sourdough	2.0%
	Deli Sourdough French Bread	2.8%
	Italian Sandwich Bread	2.9%
Freihofer	Premium Italian Sourdough	0.0%
	Brown 'N Serve Dinner Rolls	0.0%
	Family White Bread	1.0%
	Italiano Seeded Bread	1.6%
	Italiano Unseeded Bread	1.6%
	Premium Italian Bread	1.6%
	Premium Italian Seeded Bread	1.6%
	Sourdough Italiano!	1.6%
	Soft Rye No Seeds	1.7%
	Soft Rye Seeded	1.7%
	Bulkie Rolls	2.4%
	Bulkie Rolls With Seeds	2.4%
	Country White Bread	2.8%
Great Value	White Enriched Bread	1.2%
Holsum	Deli Rye Bread	2.5%
	Deli Sourdough	2.5%
Marketside	Pumpernickel Loaf Bread	1.8%
	Seeded Rye Loaf Bread	1.8%
Mestemacher	Sunflower Seed Bread	0.0%
	Whole Rye Bread	0.0%
	Fitness Bread	1.4%

Breads - alphabetical (continued)

Maker	Product	Percent Sugar
Mrs. Baird's	Sugar Free Whole Grain Wheat Bread	0.0%
Natural Valley	Light Italian Sourdough Bread	2.2%
Nature's Own	100% Whole Wheat Whole Grain Bread	0.0%
	Whole Grain Sugar Free Bread	0.0%
	40 Calorie White Bread	1.1%
	Double Fiber Wheat Bread	1.8%
	100% Whole Wheat Bread	1.9%
	Sourdough Bread	2.2%
	40 Calorie Wheat Bread	2.2%
Old London	Sourdough Melba Toast	0.0%
	Ancient Grains Melba Toast	0.0%
	Rye Melba Toast	0.0%
	Wheat Melba Toast	0.0%
	No Salt Whole Grain Melba Toast	0.0%
	Whole Grain Melba Toast	0.0%
	Classic Melba Toast	0.0%
	Rosemary & Olive Oil Melba Toast	0.0%
	Sesame Melba Toast	0.0%
Pepperidge Farm	Jewish Rye Seedless Bread	1.6%
	Deli Swirl Rye & Pump Bread	1.6%
Sara Lee	Delightful White Bread	2.2%
Seattle International	Vienna Sourdough Bread	0.0%
	French Baguette	0.0%
	Classic Sourdough Bread	0.0%

Breads - alphabetical (continued)

Maker	Product	Percent Sugar
Seattle Sourdough Baking Co.	Old Town Sourdough Bread	0.0%
	Parmesan Garlic Sourdough Bread	0.0%
	Waterfront Sourdough Bread	1.8%
Taliano	Sliced Italian Bread	0.0%
The Bakery	Seeded Rye Bread	0.8%
	Pumpernickel Bread	0.8%
Wheat Montana Farms	6 Carb, Wheat & Fibre Bread	2.9%

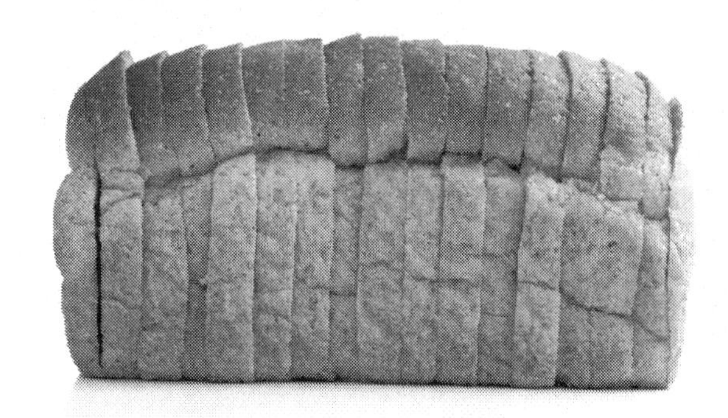

Crackers

I've presented this list in two formats so you can browse by sugar content or brand.

Most of these crackers will contain seed oils (usually soybean oil).
If you are concerned about this, then use the fat reckoner chart available at www.howmuchsugar.com to determine whether your choice is likely to be as low in seed oil as it is in sugar.

Crackers - by sugar content

Label	% Sugar
Annie's Cheddar Bunnies	0%
Beigel & Beigel Cracker Crisps Mediterranean Herbs	0%
Blue Diamond Nut Thins Cheddar Cheese	0%
Blue Diamond Nut Thins Smokehouse	0%
Blue Diamond Nut Thins Almond	0%
Blue Diamond Nut Thins Pecan	0%
Carr's Rosemary Crackers	0%
Carr's Table Water Crackers	0%
Cheez-It Asiago	0%
Cheez-It Baby Swiss	0%
Cheez-It Original	0%
Cheez-It Cheddar Jack	0%
Cheez-It Colby	0%
Cheez-It Duoz Sharp Cheddar & Parmesan	0%
Cheez-It Duoz Smoked Cheddar & Monterey Jack	0%

Crackers - by sugar content (continued)

Label	% Sugar
Cheez-It Game Day Bucket	0%
Cheez-It Gripz	0%
Cheez-It Hot & Spicy	0%
Cheez-It Four Cheese	0%
Cheez-It Monterey Jack	0%
Cheez-It Mozzarella	0%
Cheez-It Pepper Jack	0%
Cheez-It Reduced Fat	0%
Cheez-It Romano	0%
Cheez-It Scrabble Junior	0%
Cheez-It White Cheddar	0%
Cheez-It White Cheddar Reduced Fat	0%
Cheez-It Wholegrain	0%
Cheez-It Zingz Queso Fundido	0%
Crunchmaster Multigrain Crisps Original	0%
Doctor Kracker Flatbread Pumpkin Seed Cheddar	0%
Excelsior Water Crackers	0%
Great Value Snack Crackers Double Cross	0%
Great Value Cheese Crackers	0%
Kashi Heart to Heart Original	0%
Kashi Heart to Heart Roasted Garlic	0%
Keebler Town House Wheat	0%
Keebler Zesta Original	0%
Lu Water Crackers Extra Virgin Olive Oil with Sea Salt	0%
Miltons Baked Crackers Crispy Sea Salt	0%

Crackers - by sugar content (continued)

Label	% Sugar
Nabisco Saltine Original	0%
Nabisco Premium Low Sodium	0%
Nabisco Premium Original	0%
Nabisco Premium Rounds Rosemary & Olive Oil	0%
Nabisco Premium Wholegrain	0%
Nabisco Premium Unsalted Tops	0%
Nabisco Better Cheddars	0%
Nabisco Red Oval Farm Stoned Wheat Thins	0%
Nabisco Rice Thins Original	0%
Nabisco Triscuit Garden Herb	0%
Nabisco Triscuit Cracked Pepper & Olive Oil	0%
Nabisco Triscuit Dill, Sea Salt & Olive Oil	0%
Nabisco Triscuit Fire Roasted Tomato & Olive Oil	0%
Nabisco Triscuit Original	0%
Nabisco Triscuit Reduced Fat	0%
Nabisco Triscuit Roasted Garlic	0%
Nabisco Triscuit Rosemary & Olive Oil	0%
Nabisco Triscuit Hint of Salt	0%
Nabisco Triscuit Thin Crisps Original	0%
Nabisco Triscuit Brown Rice Sea Salt & Black Pepper	0%
Old London Melba Toast Classic	0%
Sunshine Krispy Wheat	0%
World Table Cheddar Jalepeno Bites	0%
World Table Sharp Cheddar Bites	0%
Pepperidge Farm Goldfish Baby	1%

Crackers - by sugar content (continued)

Label	% Sugar
Pepperidge Farm Goldfish Original	2%
Pepperidge Farm Goldfish Flavor Blasted Xplosive Pizza	2%
Stauffer's Whales	2%
Kashi TLC Zesty Salsa	3%
Nabisco Triscuit Thin Crisps Parmesan Garlic	3%
34 Degrees Crispbread Rosemary	3%
Excelsior Cheese Krunchies	3%
Excelsior Cream Crackers	3%
Kashi TLC Country Cheddar	3%
Kelloggs Special K Cracker Chips	3%
Nabisco Rice Thins Sea Salt & Pepper	3%
Nabisco Rice Thins White Cheddar	3%
Oishi Prawn Crackers Black Pepper	3%
Pepperidge Farm Goldfish Cheddar	3%
Pepperidge Farm Goldfish Colours	3%
Pepperidge Farm Goldfish Flavor Blasted Xtra Cheddar	3%
Pepperidge Farm Goldfish Wholegrain	3%
Cheez-It Zingz Chipotle Cheddar	3%
Nabisco Triscuit Brown Rice Roasted Red Pepper	3%
Nabisco Triscuit Brown Rice Savoury Red Bean	3%
Nabisco Triscuit Brown Rice Roasted Sweet Onion	3%
Nabisco Triscuit Brown Rice Tomato & Sweet Basil	3%

Crackers - alphabetical

Company	Product	Variant	% Sugar
34 Degrees	Crispbread	Rosemary	3%
Annie's	Cheddar Bunnies		0%
Beigel & Beigel	Cracker Crisps	Mediterranean Herbs	0%
Blue Diamond	Nut Thins	Cheddar Cheese	0%
	Nut Thins	Smokehouse	0%
	Nut Thins	Almond	0%
	Nut Thins	Pecan	0%
Carr's	Rosemary Crackers		0%
	Table Water Crackers		0%
Cheez-It	Asiago		0%
	Baby Swiss		0%
	Original		0%
	Cheddar Jack		0%
	Colby		0%
	Duoz	Sharp Cheddar & Parmesan	0%
	Duoz	Smoked Cheddar & Monterey Jack	0%
	Game Day Bucket		0%
	Gripz		0%
	Hot & Spicy		0%
	Four Cheese		0%
	Monterey Jack		0%
	Mozzarella		0%

Crackers - alphabetical (continued)

Company	Product	Variant	% Sugar
Cheez-It	Pepper Jack		0%
	Reduced Fat		0%
	Romano		0%
	Scrabble Junior		0%
	White Cheddar		0%
	White Cheddar	Reduced Fat	0%
	Wholegrain		0%
	Zingz	Queso Fundido	0%
	Zingz	Chipotle Cheddar	3%
Crunchmaster	Multigrain Crisps	Original	0%
Doctor Kracker	Flatbread	Pumpkin Seed Cheddar	0%
Excelsior	Water Crackers		0%
	Cheese Krunchies		3%
	Cream Crackers		3%
Great Value	Snack Crackers	Double Cross	0%
	Cheese Crackers		0%
Kashi	Heart to Heart	Original	0%
	Heart to Heart	Roasted Garlic	0%
	TLC	Zesty Salsa	3%
	TLC	Country Cheddar	3%
Keebler	Town House	Wheat	0%
	Zesta	Original	0%
Kelloggs	Special K	Cracker Chips	3%
Lu	Water Crackers	Extra Virgin Olive Oil with Sea Salt	0%

Crackers - alphabetical (continued)

Company	Product	Variant	% Sugar
Miltons	Baked Crackers	Crispy Sea Salt	0%
Nabisco	Saltine	Original	0%
	Premium	Low Sodium	0%
	Premium	Original	0%
	Premium	Rounds Rosemary & Olive Oil	0%
	Premium	Wholegrain	0%
	Premium	Unsalted Tops	0%
	Better Cheddars		0%
	Red Oval Farm	Stoned Wheat Thins	0%
	Rice Thins	Original	0%
	Triscuit	Garden Herb	0%
	Triscuit	Cracked Pepper & Olive Oil	0%
	Triscuit	Dill, Sea Salt & Olive Oil	0%
	Triscuit	Fire Roasted Tomato & Olive Oil	0%
	Triscuit	Original	0%
	Triscuit	Reduced Fat	0%
	Triscuit	Roasted Garlic	0%
	Triscuit	Rosemary & Olive Oil	0%
	Triscuit	Hint of Salt	0%
	Triscuit Thin Crisps	Original	0%
	Triscuit Brown Rice	Sea Salt & Black Pepper	0%
	Triscuit Thin Crisps	Parmesan Garlic	3%

Crackers - alphabetical (continued)

Company	Product	Variant	% Sugar
Nabisco	Rice Thins	Sea Salt & Pepper	3%
	Rice Thins	White Cheddar	3%
	Triscuit Brown Rice	Roasted Red Pepper	3%
	Triscuit Brown Rice	Savoury Red Bean	3%
	Triscuit Brown Rice	Roasted Sweet Onion	3%
	Triscuit Brown Rice	Tomato & Sweet Basil	3%
Oishi	Prawn Crackers	Black Pepper	3%
Old London	Melba Toast	Classic	0%
Pepperidge Farm	Goldfish	Baby	1%
	Goldfish	Original	2%
	Goldfish	Flavor Blasted Xplosive Pizza	2%
	Goldfish	Cheddar	3%
	Goldfish	Colours	3%
	Goldfish	Flavor Blasted Xtra Cheddar	3%
	Goldfish	Wholegrain	3%
Stauffer's	Whales		2%
Sunshine	Krispy Wheat		0%
World Table	Cheddar Jalepeno Bites		0%
	Sharp Cheddar Bites		0%

Frozen Pizza

I've presented this list in two formats so you can browse by sugar content or brand.

Most of these frozen pizzas will contain seed oils. If you are concerned about this, then use the fat reckoner chart available at www.howmuchsugar.com to determine whether your choice is likely to be as low in seed oil as it is in sugar.

Frozen Pizza - by sugar content

Pizza	% Sugar
Home Run Inn Signature Meat Lovers	0.7%
Home Run Inn Signature Sausage & Mushroom	0.7%
Home Run Inn Classic Sausage	0.7%
Home Run Inn Ultra Thin Sausage	0.7%
Home Run Inn Ultra Thin Sausage & Uncured Pepperoni	0.7%
Home Run Inn Classic Margherita	0.7%
World Table Thin Crust Buffalo Stye Chicken	0.7%
Portesi Original Style Mushroom	0.8%
Home Run Inn Classic Sausage & Uncured Pepperoni	0.8%
Home Run Inn Ultra Thin Uncured Pepperoni	0.8%
Portesi Original Style Sausage	0.8%
Sam's Choice Flatbread Loaded Baked Potato	0.8%
Home Run Inn Ultra Thin Cheese	0.9%
Home Run Inn Classic Cheese	0.9%
Tombstone Mini Pizza Pepperoni	1.1%
Michael Angelo's Flat Bread Mediterranean	1.2%
Michael Angelo's Flat Bread Pepperoni & Salami	1.2%
Home Run Inn Signature Sausage Supreme with Fireroasted Vegetables	1.3%

Frozen Pizza - by sugar content (continued)

Pizza	% Sugar
Sam's Choice Thin Crust Supreme	1.3%
Portesi Original Style Cheese & Sausage	1.3%
Marketside Traditional Crust Philly Cheesesteak	1.3%
Roma Deluxe	1.4%
DiGiorno Pizza Dipping Strips Three Meat	1.4%
World Table Thin Crust Philly Cheesesteak	1.5%
California Pizza Kitchen Crispy Thin Crust Garlic Chicken	1.5%
DiGiorno Pizza Dipping Strips Pepperoni	1.5%
Orv's Ultimate Rizer Special Deluxe	1.5%
California Pizza Kitchen Crispy Thin Crust Chicken Carbonara	1.5%
DiGiorno Crispy Flatbread Tuscan Style Chicken	1.5%
DiGiorno Pizza Dipping Strips Four Cheese	1.5%
Freschetta Flat Bread Zesty Italian Style	1.5%
DiGiorno Pizzeria! Bianca	1.6%
California Pizza Kitchen Crispy Thin Crust White	1.6%
Red Baron French Bread 5 Cheese & Garlic	1.6%
Roma Sausage	1.6%
Roma 3 meat	1.6%
California Pizza Kitchen Crispy Thin Crust Margherita	1.7%
Freschetta Flat Bread 5 Cheese	1.7%
Marketside Traditional Crust Tuscan Vegetable	1.7%
Sam's Choice Flatbread Chicken Spinach Mushroom	1.7%
Sam's Choice Flatbread Chicken Chipotle	1.7%
Freschetta Flat Bread Pepperoni	1.7%
Freschetta Flat Bread Roasted Garlic & Spinach	1.7%

Frozen Pizza - by sugar content (continued)

Pizza	% Sugar
DiGiorno Thin & Crispy Spinach & Garlic	1.8%
Gino's East of Chicago Deep Dish Sausage	1.8%
Gino's East of Chicago Deep Dish Cheese	1.8%
Gino's East of Chicago Deep Dish Spinach & Garlic	1.8%
Gino's East of Chicago Deep Dish Sausage Patty	1.8%
Green Mill Thin N Crispy Style Il primo	1.8%
Great Value Fully Loaded Pepperoni	1.9%
DiGiorno Crispy Flatbread Italian Sausage & Onions	1.9%
Fresh Bake by Donato's Thin Crust Pepperoni & Sausage	1.9%
Palermo's Primo Thin Grillen Chicken Caesar	2.0%
Green Mill Thin N Crispy Style Triple Meat	2.0%
Orv's Ultimate Rizer Three Meat	2.0%
Tony's Pizza for One Pepperoni	2.0%
Fresh Bake by Donato's Thin Crust Pepperoni	2.1%
Sam's Choice Thin Crust Chicken Bacon Ranch	2.1%
Celeste Pizza for One Original	2.1%
Orv's Ultimate Rizer Extra Cheese	2.1%
Tombstone Double Top Classic Sausage	2.1%
Great Value Thin Crust Cheese	2.1%
Totino's Party Pizza Mexican Style	2.1%
DiGiorno Original Thin Crust Supreme	2.1%
DiGiorno 200 Calorie Portions Chicken with Peppers & Onions	2.1%
DiGiorno Crispy Flatbread Supreme	2.2%
Newman's Own Thin & Crispy Supreme	2.2%
Tony's Pizza for One Cheese	2.2%
Portesi Thin Crust Mushroom	2.2%

Frozen Pizza - by sugar content (continued)

Pizza	% Sugar
Sam's Choice Thin Crust Pepperoni	2.2%
Lean Cuisine Deep Dish Spincah & Artichoke	2.2%
Palermo's Primo Thin Italian Sausage	2.2%
Palermo's Primo Thin Sicilian	2.2%
Tombstone Double Top Pepperoni	2.2%
DiGiorno Pizzeria! Primo Pepperoni	2.3%
DiGiorno Original Thin Crust Four Meat	2.3%
Palermo's Hand Tossed Style Supreme	2.3%
Stouffer's French Bread Three Meat	2.3%
Palermo's Original Thin Crust Sausage & Mushroom	2.3%
Sam's Choice Flatbread Nacho Supreme	2.3%
DiGiorno Crispy Flatbread Fire Roasted Peppers, Tomato & Spinach	2.3%
DiGiorno Pizzeria! Four Cheese	2.3%
DiGiorno Original Thin Crust Four Cheese	2.3%
Tombstone Double Top 4 Meat	2.3%
Orv's Ultimate Rizer Sausage & Mushroom	2.3%
Roma Supreme	2.3%
California Pizza Kitchen Crispy Thin Crust Signature Pepperoni	2.3%
Gino's East of Chicago Thin Crust Sausage & Pepperoni	2.3%
Gino's East of Chicago Thin Crust Sausage	2.3%
Great Value Thin Crust Supreme	2.3%
Orv's Ultimate Rizer Pepperoni Supreme	2.3%
Michael Angelo's Flat Bread Saausage & Mushroom	2.4%
California Pizza Kitchen Crispy Thin Crust Four Cheese	2.4%
Newman's Own Thin & Crispy Four Cheese	2.4%

Frozen Pizza - by sugar content (continued)

Pizza	% Sugar
Stouffer's French Bread Extra Cheese	2.4%
DiGiorno Original Thin Crust Pepperoni	2.4%
Newman's Own Thin & Crispy Uncured Pepperoni	2.4%
Palermo's Hand Tossed Style Italian Sausage	2.4%
Portesi Thin Crust Cheese & Sausage	2.4%
Amy's Kitchen Margherita	2.4%
Freschetta California-Style Bacon, Spinach & artichoke	2.4%
Freschetta California-Style Mediterranean Garlic Veggie	2.4%
Red Baron French Bread Supreme	2.4%
Roma Bacon Cheeseburger	2.4%
Great Value Thin Crust Sausage & Pepperoni	2.5%
DiGiorno Thin & Crispy Tomato Mozzarella with Pesto	2.5%
Orv's Tasty Toppings Sausage Supreme	2.5%
Tony's Original Crust Sausage	2.5%
Totino's Party Pizza Combination	2.5%
Celeste Pizza for One Vegetable	2.5%
Orv's Tasty Toppings Veggie Supreme	2.5%
Stouffer's French Bread Pepperoni	2.5%
DiGiorno Crispy Flatbread Italian Three Cheese	2.5%
Orv's Tasty Toppings Pepperoni Supreme	2.5%
Red Baron French Bread 3 Meat	2.6%
Totino's Party Pizza Hamburger	2.6%
Totino's Party Pizza Supreme	2.6%
Reser's Fine Foods Deluxe Combo	2.6%
Red Baron French Bread Pepperoni	2.6%

Frozen Pizza - by sugar content (continued)

Pizza	% Sugar
Tombstone Double Top Supreme	2.6%
Totino's Party Pizza Sausage	2.6%
Celeste Pizza for One Sausage	2.6%
Tombstone Original Pepperoni & Sausage	2.6%
DiGiorno Pizzeria! Supreme	2.6%
Tombstone Garlic Dipping Bites Supreme	2.6%
Totino's Party Pizza Cheese	2.6%
DiGiorno Thin & Crispy Pepperoni & Peppers	2.7%
Palermo's Hand Tossed Style Combination	2.7%
Totino's Party Pizza Triple Meat	2.7%
California Pizza Kitchen Crispy Thin Crust Sicilian recipe	2.7%
Stouffer's French Bread Cheese	2.7%
Totino's Party Pizza Canadian Style Bacon	2.7%
DiGiorno Pizzeria! Italian Meat Trio	2.8%
Great Value Fully Loaded Mega Meat	2.8%
Totino's Party Pizza Pepperoni	2.8%
Totino's Party Pizza triple Pepperoni	2.8%
World Table Thin Crust Pepperoni with Fresh Mozzarella	2.8%
Palermo's Hand Tossed Style Pepperoni	2.8%
Tombstone Garlic Dipping Bites Pepperoni	2.8%
Tombstone Garlic Dipping Bites Cheese	2.8%
Stouffer's French Bread Sausage & Pepperoni	2.8%
DiGiorno Deep Dish Italian Sausage	2.8%
Jeno's Crisp N Tasty Cheese	2.8%
Jack's Pizza Fries	2.9%

Frozen Pizza - by sugar content (continued)

Pizza	% Sugar
Stouffer's French Bread Deluxe	2.9%
Great Value Fully Loaded Double Pepperoni	2.9%
Totino's Party Pizza Classic Pepperoni	2.9%
Lean Cuisine Deep Dish Spinach & Mushroom	2.9%
Weight Watchers Artisan Creation Stone Fired Pepperoni	2.9%
Great Value Fully Loaded Chicken Bacon & Ranch	2.9%
Palermo's Original Thin Crust Deluxe	2.9%
Totino's Party Pizza Triple Cheese	2.9%
Palermo's Hand Tossed Style Cheese	2.9%
Tombstone Brick Oven Style Supreme	2.9%
California Pizza Kitchen Crispy Thin Crust Fire Roasted Vegetables	3.0%
California Pizza Kitchen Crispy Thin Crust Chipotle Roasted Vegetables	3.0%
Jack's Original Mexican Style	3.0%
Great Value Rising Crust Four Cheese	3.0%
Amy's Kitchen Spinach	3.0%
Roma Sausage & Mushroom	3.0%

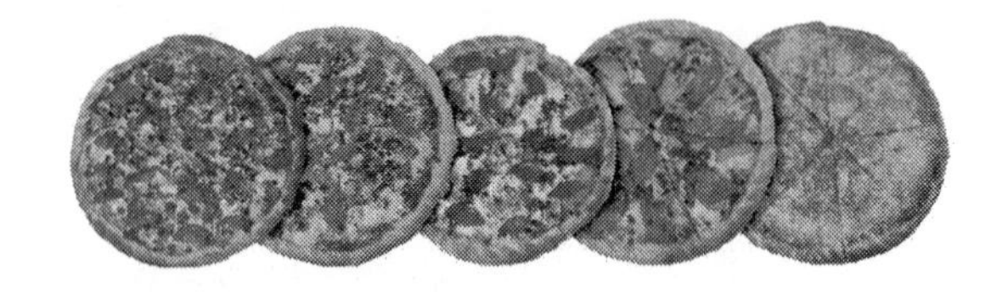

Frozen Pizza - alphabetical

Brand	Item	Sub-Item	% Sugar
Amy's Kitchen	Margherita		2.4%
	Spinach		3.0%
California Pizza Kitchen	Crispy Thin Crust	Garlic Chicken	1.5%
	Crispy Thin Crust	Chicken Carbonara	1.5%
	Crispy Thin Crust	White	1.6%
	Crispy Thin Crust	Margherita	1.7%
	Crispy Thin Crust	Signature Pepperoni	2.3%
	Crispy Thin Crust	Four Cheese	2.4%
	Crispy Thin Crust	Sicilian recipe	2.7%
	Crispy Thin Crust	Fire Roasted Vegetables	3.0%
	Crispy Thin Crust	Chipotle Roasted Vegetables	3.0%
Celeste	Pizza for One	Original	2.1%
	Pizza for One	Vegetable	2.5%
	Pizza for One	Sausage	2.6%
DiGiorno	Pizza Dipping Strips	Three Meat	1.4%
	Pizza Dipping Strips	Pepperoni	1.5%
	Crispy Flatbread	Tuscan Style Chicken	1.5%
	Pizza Dipping Strips	Four Cheese	1.5%
	Pizzeria!	Bianca	1.6%
	Thin & Crispy	Spinach & Garlic	1.8%
	Crispy Flatbread	Italian Sausage & Onions	1.9%
	Original Thin Crust	Supreme	2.1%
	200 Calorie Portions	Chicken with Peppers & Onions	2.1%

Frozen Pizza - alphabetical (continued)

Brand	Item	Sub-Item	% Sugar
DiGiorno	Crispy Flatbread	Supreme	2.2%
	Pizzeria!	Primo Pepperoni	2.3%
	Original Thin Crust	Four Meat	2.3%
	Crispy Flatbread	Fire Roasted Peppers, Tomato & Spinach	2.3%
	Pizzeria!	Four Cheese	2.3%
	Original Thin Crust	Four Cheese	2.3%
	Original Thin Crust	Pepperoni	2.4%
	Thin & Crispy	Tomato Mozzarella with Pesto	2.5%
	Crispy Flatbread	Italian Three Cheese	2.5%
	Pizzeria!	Supreme	2.6%
	Thin & Crispy	Pepperoni & Peppers	2.7%
	Pizzeria!	Italian Meat Trio	2.8%
	Deep Dish	Italian Sausage	2.8%
Freschetta	Flat Bread	Zesty Italian Style	1.5%
	Flat Bread	5 Cheese	1.7%
	Flat Bread	Pepperoni	1.7%
	Flat Bread	Roasted Garlic & Spinach	1.7%
	California-Style	Bacon, Spinach & artichoke	2.4%
	California-Style	Mediterranean Garlic Veggie	2.4%
Fresh Bake by Donato's	Thin Crust	Pepperoni & Sausage	1.9%
	Thin Crust	Pepperoni	2.1%
Gino's East of Chicago	Deep Dish	Sausage	1.8%

Frozen Pizza - alphabetical (continued)

Brand	Item	Sub-Item	% Sugar
Gino's East of Chicago	Deep Dish	Cheese	1.8%
	Deep Dish	Spinach & Garlic	1.8%
	Deep Dish	Sausage Patty	1.8%
	Thin Crust	Sausage & Pepperoni	2.3%
	Thin Crust	Sausage	2.3%
Great Value	Fully Loaded	Pepperoni	1.9%
	Thin Crust	Cheese	2.1%
	Thin Crust	Supreme	2.3%
	Thin Crust	Sausage & Pepperoni	2.5%
	Fully Loaded	Mega Meat	2.8%
	Fully Loaded	Double Pepperoni	2.9%
	Fully Loaded	Chicken Bacon & Ranch	2.9%
	Rising Crust	Four Cheese	3.0%
Green Mill	Thin N Crispy Style	Il primo	1.8%
	Thin N Crispy Style	Triple Meat	2.0%
Home Run Inn	Signature	Meat Lovers	0.7%
	Signature	Sausage & Mushroom	0.7%
	Classic	Sausage	0.7%
	Ultra Thin	Sausage	0.7%
	Ultra Thin	Sausage & Uncured Pepperoni	0.7%
	Classic	Margherita	0.7%
	Classic	Sausage & Uncured Pepperoni	0.8%
	Ultra Thin	Uncured Pepperoni	0.8%

Frozen Pizza - alphabetical (continued)

Brand	Item	Sub-Item	% Sugar
Home Run Inn	Ultra Thin	Cheese	0.9%
	Classic	Cheese	0.9%
	Signature	Sausage Supreme with Fireroasted Vegetables	1.3%
Jack's	Pizza Fries		2.9%
	Original	Mexican Style	3.0%
	Crisp N Tasty	Cheese	2.8%
Lean Cuisine	Deep Dish	Spincah & Artichoke	2.2%
	Deep Dish	Spinach & Mushroom	2.9%
Marketside	Traditional Crust	Philly Cheesesteak	1.3%
	Traditional Crust	Tuscan Vegetable	1.7%
Michael Angelo's	Flat Bread	Mediterranean	1.2%
	Flat Bread	Pepperoni & Salami	1.2%
	Flat Bread	Saausage & Mushroom	2.4%
Newman's Own	Thin & Crispy	Supreme	2.2%
	Thin & Crispy	Four Cheese	2.4%
	Thin & Crispy	Uncured Pepperoni	2.4%
Orv's	Ultimate Rizer	Special Deluxe	1.5%
	Ultimate Rizer	Three Meat	2.0%
	Ultimate Rizer	Extra Cheese	2.1%
	Ultimate Rizer	Sausage & Mushroom	2.3%
	Ultimate Rizer	Pepperoni Supreme	2.3%
	Tasty Toppings	Sausage Supreme	2.5%

Frozen Pizza - alphabetical (continued)

Brand	Item	Sub-Item	% Sugar
Orv's	Tasty Toppings	Veggie Supreme	2.5%
	Tasty Toppings	Pepperoni Supreme	2.5%
Palermo's	Primo Thin	Grillen Chicken Caesar	2.0%
	Primo Thin	Italian Sausage	2.2%
	Primo Thin	Sicilian	2.2%
	Hand Tossed Style	Supreme	2.3%
	Original Thin Crust	Sausage & Mushroom	2.3%
	Hand Tossed Style	Italian Sausage	2.4%
	Hand Tossed Style	Combination	2.7%
	Hand Tossed Style	Pepperoni	2.8%
	Original Thin Crust	Deluxe	2.9%
	Hand Tossed Style	Cheese	2.9%
Portesi	Original Style	Mushroom	0.8%
	Original Style	Sausage	0.8%
	Original Style	Cheese & Sausage	1.3%
	Thin Crust	Mushroom	2.2%
	Thin Crust	Cheese & Sausage	2.4%
Red Baron	French Bread	5 Cheese & Garlic	1.6%
	French Bread	Supreme	2.4%
	French Bread	3 Meat	2.6%
	French Bread	Pepperoni	2.6%
Reser's Fine Foods	Deluxe Combo		2.6%
Roma	Deluxe		1.4%
	Sausage		1.6%

Frozen Pizza - alphabetical (continued)

Brand	Item	Sub-Item	% Sugar
Roma	3 meat		1.6%
	Supreme		2.3%
	Bacon Cheeseburger		2.4%
	Sausage & Mushroom	3.0%	
Sam's Choice	Flatbread	Loaded Baked Potato	0.8%
	Thin Crust	Supreme	1.3%
	Flatbread	Chicken Spinach Mushroom	1.7%
	Flatbread	Chicken Chipotle	1.7%
	Thin Crust	Chicken Bacon Ranch	2.1%
	Thin Crust	Pepperoni	2.2%
	Flatbread	Nacho Supreme	2.3%
Stouffer's	French Bread	Three Meat	2.3%
	French Bread	Extra Cheese	2.4%
	French Bread	Pepperoni	2.5%
	French Bread	Cheese	2.7%
	French Bread	Sausage & Pepperoni	2.8%
	French Bread	Deluxe	2.9%
Tombstone	Mini Pizza	Pepperoni	1.1%
	Double Top	Classic Sausage	2.1%
	Double Top	Pepperoni	2.2%
	Double Top	4 Meat	2.3%
	Double Top	Supreme	2.6%
	Original	Pepperoni & Sausage	2.6%
	Garlic Dipping Bites	Supreme	2.6%

Frozen Pizza - alphabetical (continued)

Brand	Item	Sub-Item	% Sugar
Tombstone	Garlic Dipping Bites	Pepperoni	2.8%
	Garlic Dipping Bites	Cheese	2.8%
	Brick Oven Style	Supreme	2.9%
Tony's	Pizza for One	Pepperoni	2.0%
	Pizza for One	Cheese	2.2%
	Original Crust	Sausage	2.5%
Totino's	Party Pizza	Mexican Style	2.1%
	Party Pizza	Combination	2.5%
	Party Pizza	Hamburger	2.6%
	Party Pizza	Supreme	2.6%
	Party Pizza	Sausage	2.6%
	Party Pizza	Cheese	2.6%
	Party Pizza	Triple Meat	2.7%
	Party Pizza	Canadian Style Bacon	2.7%
	Party Pizza	Pepperoni	2.8%
	Party Pizza	triple Pepperoni	2.8%
	Party Pizza	Classic Pepperoni	2.9%
	Party Pizza	Triple Cheese	2.9%
Weight Watchers	Artisan Creation	Stone Fired Pepperoni	2.9%
World Table	Thin Crust	Buffalo Stye Chicken	0.7%
	Thin Crust	Philly Cheesesteak	1.5%
	Thin Crust	Pepperoni with Fresh Mozzarella	2.8%

Frozen Dinners

I've presented this list in two formats so you can browse by sugar content or brand.

Most of these frozen dinners will contain seed oils. If you are concerned about this, then use the fat reckoner chart available at www.howmuchsugar.com to determine whether your choice is likely to be as low in seed oil as it is in sugar.

Frozen Dinners - by sugar content

Dinner	% sugar
Albie's Chicken Pasties	0.0%
Chaparro's Beef Tamales	0.0%
Chaparro's Pork Tamales	0.0%
El Cazo Mexicano Beef Tamales	0.0%
Gardenburger The original Veggie burgers	0.0%
Hanover Caribbean Black Beans in Sauce Bean Essentials	0.0%
Herdez Carnitas & Charro Beans Bowl Cocina Mexicana	0.0%
Jimmy Dean Bacon Breakfast Bowl	0.0%
Jimmy Dean Sausage Breakfast Bowl	0.0%
Marie Callender's Braised Beef Pot Roast Comfort Bakes	0.0%
Marie Callender's Savory Chicken & Rice Comfort Bakes	0.0%
McKenzie's Southern Field Peas With Snaps	0.0%
Morning Star Farms Mushroom Lover's Veggie burgers	0.0%
Night Hawk Charbroiled bites & Taters	0.0%
Night Hawk Steak 'N Taters	0.0%
Owens Sausage Biscuits Snackwiches	0.0%

Frozen Dinners - by sugar content (continued)

Dinner	% sugar
Snapps Cheese Sticks Snackbites	0.0%
T.G.I. Friday's Buffalo Style Sauce Boneless Chicken Bites	0.0%
Weight Watchers Chicken Strips & Fries Smart Ones	0.0%
Weight Watchers Slow Roasted Turkey Breast Smart Ones	0.0%
El Charrito Mexican Style Enchiladas Grande	0.2%
El Charrito Beef echiladas Meal for Two	0.3%
An-Joy Chicken Fried Rice	0.4%
Herdez Pork Chile Colorado Bowl Cocina Mexicana	0.4%
Zatarain With Beef & Pork Dirty Rice	0.4%
Atkins Chicken & Broccoli Alfredo	0.4%
Healthy Choice Fettuccini Alfredo Bake Baked	0.4%
Banquet Southwestern style patty	0.4%
Jimmy Dean Sausage & gravy Breakfast bowl	0.4%
Michelina's Salisbury Steak Traditional	0.4%
Marie Callender's Egg Cheese & Ham Bake Breakfast Anytime	0.4%
Banquet Creamy Sauce With Broccoli & Chicken Over Rice Family size	0.5%
Marie Callender's Cheesy Egg & Sausage Bake Breakfast Anytime	0.5%
Marie Callender's Meat Loaf & Gravy	0.5%
Marie Callender's Turkey Breast & Stuffing	0.5%
Banquet Fettucine Alfredo	0.5%
Savoie's Eggs, Andouille & Potatoes with Gravy Cajun Daybreak	0.5%
Marie Callender's Chunky Chicken & noodles	0.5%
Weight Watchers Ham and Cheese Scramble Smart Ones	0.5%

Frozen Dinners - by sugar content (continued)

Dinner	% sugar
El Charrito Saltillo enchilada dinner Grande	0.6%
Bertolli Steak Rigatoni & Portabello Mushrooms Mediterranean style	0.6%
Richard's Cajun Favourites Seafood Jambalaya	0.6%
Richard's Cajun Favourites Shrimp Etouffee	0.6%
Stouffer's Escalloped Chicken & Noodles Classics	0.6%
Tai Pei Chicken fried rice	0.6%
Zatarain Chicken & Sausage Jambalaya Meal For Two	0.6%
Zatarain Smothered Chicken & Rice Meal For Two	0.6%
Pagoda Express Chicken Fried Rice	0.6%
Barefoot Contessa Jambalaya	0.6%
Marie Callender's Penne Chicken Modesto Pasta al dente	0.6%
Marie Callender's Country Fried Chicken & Gravy	0.7%
Michael Angelo's Chicken Piccata	0.7%
Banquet Chicken nuggets and fries	0.7%
El Charrito Beef & Cheese Rolled Tacos	0.7%
Michelina's Pop'n Chicken Traditional	0.7%
Herdez Beef Barbacoa Bowl Cocina Mexicana	0.7%
Herdez Chicken Chipotle Bowl Cocina Mexicana	0.7%
Herdez Huevos Rancheros Bowl Cocina Mexicana	0.7%
Marie Callender's Cheddar & Bacon Potato Bake Comfort Bakes	0.7%
Marie Callender's Chicken & Broccoli Alfredo Comfort Bakes	0.7%
Savoie's Chicken & Sausage Jambalaya Cajun Singles	0.7%
Stouffer's Braised Beef & Roasted Red Skin Potatoes Satisfying Servings	0.7%

Frozen Dinners - by sugar content (continued)

Dinner	% sugar
Barber Foods Cheddar Jalepeno Stuffed chicken breasts	0.7%
Barber Foods Loaded Baked Potato Stuffed chicken breasts	0.7%
Barber Foods Pot Pie Taste Stuffed chicken breasts	0.7%
Barber Foods Broccoli & Cheese Stuffed chicken breasts	0.7%
Boston Market Beef Steak & Pasta Homestyle Meals	0.8%
Boston Market Buffalo Style Chicken Strips with Macaroni & Cheese Homestyle Meals	0.8%
Weight Watchers Chicken Fettuccini Smart Ones	0.8%
Gluten Free Café Lemon Basil Chicken	0.8%
Hanover Tuscan White Beans in Sauce Bean Essentials	0.8%
Culinary Delights Shrimp & sauasage jambalaya Cajun Style Selections	0.8%
Banquet 6 Salisbury steaks & brown gravy	0.8%
Quirch Foods Jerk Chicken Jamaican Style Patties	0.8%
Southern Belle Lobster Mac-N-Cheese	0.8%
Atkins Crustless Chicken Pot Pie	0.8%
Atkins Meatloaf With Portebello Mushroom Gravy	0.8%
Atkins Shrimp Scampi	0.8%
Atkins Swedish Meatballs	0.8%
Stouffer's Fish Fillet Classics	0.8%
Weight Watchers Creamy Rigatoni with Broccoli & Chicken Smart Ones	0.8%
Weight Watchers Meatloaf Smart Ones	0.8%
Weight Watchers Roast Beef, Mashed Potatoes and Gravy Smart Ones	0.8%
Weight Watchers Salisbury Steak Smart Ones	0.8%
Jimmy Dean Sausage Skillets	0.8%

Frozen Dinners - by sugar content (continued)

Dinner	% sugar
Healthy Choice Chicken Enchilada Bake Baked	0.8%
Stouffer's Escalloped Chicken & Noodles Family	0.8%
Boston Market Chicken, Broccoli & Cheese Casserole Homestyle Meals	0.8%
Boston Market Turkey Breast Medallions Homestyle Meals	0.8%
Healthy Choice Chicken & Rice Cheddar Bake Baked	0.8%
Marie Callender's Cheesy Chicken & Rice Comfort Bakes	0.8%
Louisa Sausage & Cheese Toasted Ravioli	0.8%
Lean Cuisine Grilled Chicken Caesar Culinary Collection	0.8%
Michelina's Sante Fe style rice & beans Lean Gourmet	0.8%
Green Giant Cheesy Rice & Broccoli Just for One	0.8%
Healthy Choice Chicken & Spinach Alfredo Baked	0.8%
Stouffer's Rigatoni Pasta with Roasted White Meat Chicken Classics	0.8%
Culinary Delights Shrimp Etouffee Cajun Style Selections	0.9%
Don Miguel Mexican Style Lasagne Gourmet	0.9%
Mrs T's Potato & onion Pierogies	0.9%
Banquet Salisbury Steak In Gravy With Potatoes And Vegetables Family size	0.9%
Banquet Pepper steak	0.9%
Marie Callender's Vermont white cheddar mac & cheese	0.9%
Marie Callender's Creamy Chicken alfredo with sundried tomatoes	0.9%
Michelina's Macaroni & cheese	0.9%
Michelina's Sante Fe style rice & beans	0.9%
Michelina's Wheels & Cheese Pasta	0.9%
Michelina's Buffalo-Style Chicken Mac & Cheese	0.9%

Frozen Dinners - by sugar content (continued)

Dinner	% sugar
Michelina's Broccoli Cheese Chicken Lean Gourmet	0.9%
Michelina's Chicken Asiago Lean Gourmet	0.9%
Michelina's Creamy rigatoni with broccoli & chicken Lean Gourmet	0.9%
Michelina's Three cheese chicken Lean Gourmet	0.9%
Michelina's Stir fry rice & vegetables with chicken Lean Gourmet	0.9%
Michelina's Chicken Fried Rice Traditional	0.9%
Bertolli Chicken Florentine & Farfalle Classic meal for 4	0.9%
Boston Market Meatloaf & Potatoes Homestyle Bowl	0.9%
Boston Market Southwest Style Chicken With Rice Homestyle Bowl	0.9%
Great Value Shrimp Scampi & Linguini	0.9%
Stouffer's Savory Chicken & Rice Skillet	0.9%
Zatarain Flavored With Sausage Jambalaya	0.9%
Zatarain Beef & Mushroom Pasta Meal For Two	0.9%
Zatarain Sausage & Chicken Gumbo With Rice	0.9%
Stouffer's Roast Turkey Breast Satisfying Servings	0.9%
Culinary Delights Shrimp Linguini Cajun Style Selections	0.9%
Treasures from the Sea Butter Herb Shrimp	0.9%
Night Hawk Top Chop't Classic	0.9%
Lean Cuisine Steak Portabello Culinary Collection	0.9%
Richard's Cajun Favourites Crawfish Etouffee	1.0%
Boston Market Salisbury Steak Homestyle Meals	1.0%
Zatarain With Yellow Rice Blackened Chicken	1.0%
Marie Callender's Steak & Roasted Potatoes	1.0%

Frozen Dinners - by sugar content (continued)

Dinner	% sugar
T.G.I. Friday's Cheddar & Bacon Potato Skins	1.0%
Rice Gourmet Chicken Fried Rice	1.1%
Healthy Choice Roasted Chicken and Potatoes Baked	1.1%
Stouffer's Roast Turkey Classics	1.1%
On-Cor Chicken Fettucine Alfredo	1.1%
Weight Watchers Salisbury Steak Smart Ones	1.1%
Marie Callender's Scalloped Potatoes with Ham	1.1%
Snapps Loaded potato sticks Snackbites	1.1%
Stouffer's Broccoli & Beef Skillet Easy Express	1.1%
Ore-Ida Shredded Hash Brown Potatoes	1.1%
Ore-Ida Tater Tots	1.2%
Atkins Beef Merlot	1.2%
Atkins Chicken Marsala	1.2%
Atkins Italian Sausage Primavera	1.2%
Atkins Orange Chicken	1.2%
Atkins Roast Turkey Tenders With Herb Pan Gravy	1.2%
Atkins Sesame Chicken Stir-Fry	1.2%
Banquet Loaded Potato Bites	1.2%
Banquet Mac & Cheese Bites	1.2%
Bertolli Garlic Shrimp Risotto Classic meal for 2	1.2%
Bertolli Chicken Alfredo & Penne Classic meal for 3	1.2%
Boston Market Country Fried Chicken & Potatoes Homestyle Bowl	1.2%
Boston Market Beef Pot Roast Homestyle Meals	1.2%
Contessa Empanadas Fish	1.2%

Frozen Dinners - by sugar content (continued)

Dinner	% sugar
Lean Cuisine Lemon Pepper fish Culinary Collection	1.2%
Mrs T's Potato & onion mini Pierogies	1.2%
Newman's Own Chicken Florentine & Farfalle Complete Skillet Meal for Two	1.2%
Newman's Own Chicken Parmigiana & Penne Complete Skillet Meal for Two	1.2%
Newman's Own Italian Sausage & Rigatoni Complete Skillet Meal for Two	1.2%
Ore-Ida Potatoes O'Brien with Onions & Peppers	1.2%
Richard's Cajun Favourites Chicken Fettucine	1.2%
Richard's Cajun Favourites Pork & Sausage Jambalaya	1.2%
Stouffer's Macaroni & Cheese Broccoli Classics	1.2%
Stouffer's Chicken Fettuccini Alfredo Satisfying Servings	1.2%
Stouffer's Braised beef & portebello tortellini Sautes for Two	1.2%
T.G.I. Friday's Cheese & Bacon Loaded Fries	1.2%
Weight Watchers Chicken Oriental Smart Ones	1.2%
Weight Watchers Three Cheese Ziti Marinara Smart Ones	1.2%
Weight Watchers Beef Pot Roast Smart Ones	1.2%
Culinary Delights Shrimp Creole Cajun Style Selections	1.2%
Barber Foods Long Grain And Wild Rice Premium Entrees	1.2%
Gia Russa Stuffed rigatoni	1.2%
Gia Russa Tri-Colored Tortellini	1.2%
Ore-Ida Seasoned Crinkles Extra Crispy	1.2%
Ore-Ida Fast Food Fries Extra Crispy	1.2%
Ore-Ida Golden Crinkles Extra Crispy	1.2%
Ore-Ida Golden fries	1.2%

Frozen Dinners - by sugar content (continued)

Dinner	% sugar
Ore-Ida Shoestrings	1.2%
Ore-Ida Waffle Fries	1.2%
Ore-Ida Zesties	1.2%
Ore-Ida Zesty Twirls	1.2%
Stouffer's Baked Chicken Breast Classics	1.2%
Stouffer's Beef Pot Roast Classics	1.2%
Night Hawk Beef Patty 'N Gravy	1.2%
Stouffer's Cheesy Chicken & Broccoli Rice Bake	1.2%
Stouffer's Grilled Chicken & Asiago Tortellini Sautes for Two	1.2%
Stouffer's Chicken a la King Classics	1.2%
Banquet Zesty smothered meat patty	1.2%
Morning Star Farms Veggie meatballs	1.3%
Snapps Cheeseburger Fritters	1.3%
Marie Callender's Salisbury steak	1.3%
Stouffer's Savory Beef & Vegetables Satisfying Servings	1.3%
Barefoot Contessa Beef stew Bourgignon	1.3%
Barefoot Contessa Pasta carbonara with pancetta	1.3%
Barefoot Contessa Tequila lime chicken	1.3%
Stouffer's Garlic shrimp skillet Easy Express	1.3%
Stouffer's Meatloaf	1.3%
Culinary Delights Creole style paella Cajun Style Selections	1.3%
Boston Market Chicken pot pie	1.3%
Michelina's Cheeseburger Mac	1.3%
Michelina's Chicken alfredo florentine Lean Gourmet	1.3%
Michelina's Chipotle Chicken & Rice Lean Gourmet	1.3%

Frozen Dinners - by sugar content (continued)

Dinner	% sugar
Michelina's Beef & Peppers Traditional	1.3%
Michelina's White Turkey in Cream Sauce with Pasta Traditional	1.3%
Stouffer's Salisbury Steak Satisfying Servings	1.3%
Weight Watchers Chicken Fajitas Smart Ones	1.3%
Weight Watchers Steak Fajitas Smart Ones	1.3%
Gia Russa Manicotti With Ricotta Cheese	1.3%
Boston Market Country Fried Beef Steak Homestyle Meals	1.3%
Boston Market Chicken Alfredo with Fettuccine & Broccoli Homestyle Meals	1.4%
Birds Eye Chicken Florentine Voila	1.4%
Amy's Vegetable Pie	1.4%
Koch Foods Cordon Bleu Oven Cravers	1.4%
Marie Callender's Turkey pot pie	1.4%
Michelina's Meatloaf Lean Gourmet	1.4%
Morning Star Farms original Chik Veggie patties	1.4%
Stouffer's Homestyle Beef Skillet	1.4%
Herdez Pork al Pastor Bowl Cocina Mexicana	1.4%
Night Hawk Beef Patty 'N Mashed Potatoes	1.4%
Stouffer's Grilled Asiago Chicken & Penne Pasta Satisfying Servings	1.4%
Marie Callender's Mac and Cheese	1.4%
Stouffer's Rigatoni with Chicken & Pesto Family	1.4%
Tai Pei Shrimp Fried rice	1.4%
Bertolli Ricotta & Spinach Cannelloni Rustico Bakes	1.5%
Bertolli Shrimp Scampi & Linguine Classic meal for 5	1.5%

Frozen Dinners - by sugar content (continued)

Dinner	% sugar
Bertolli Shrimp, Asparagus & Penne Classic meal for 6	1.5%
Bertolli Grilled Chicken & Roasted Vegetables Mediterranean style	1.5%
Boston Market Turkey Breast & Potatoes Homestyle Bowl	1.5%
Great Value Grilled Chicken Alfredo	1.5%
Marie Callender's Golden battered fish fillet	1.5%
Night Hawk Taste of texas	1.5%
Owens Sausage Egg & Cheese Tacos Border Breakfasts	1.5%
Stouffer's Turkey Tetrazzini Classics	1.5%
Stouffer's Chicken & Dumplings Skillet	1.5%
Tai Pei Chicken Chow Mein	1.5%
Zatarain With Sausage Red Beans & Rice	1.5%
Amy's Black Bean Vegetable Enchilada	1.5%
Morning Star Farms Mediterranean Chickpea Veggie burgers	1.5%
Morning Star Farms Roasted Garlic & Quinoa Veggie burgers	1.5%
Morning Star Farms Spicy Black Bean Veggie burgers	1.5%
Great Value Chicken Enchilada Casserole	1.5%
Stouffer's Savory Beef & Vegetables	1.5%
Albie's Beef Pasties	1.5%
Boston Market Meatloaf Homestyle Meals	1.5%
Banquet Chicken and broccoli pot pie	1.5%
Bertolli Chicken Portabello Ravioli Rustico Bakes	1.5%
Stouffer's Swedish Meatballs Classics	1.5%
Hanover Cajun Pink Beans in Sauce Bean Essentials	1.5%
Hanover Southwestern Pinto Beans in Sauce Bean Essentials	1.5%

Frozen Dinners - by sugar content (continued)

Dinner	% sugar
Morning Star Farms California Turk'y Grillers	1.6%
Amy's Tofu Scramble Entrée	1.6%
Atkins Italian Style Pasta Bake	1.6%
Atkins Mexican Style Chicken And Vegetables	1.6%
Lean Cuisine Chicken Fried Rice Simple Favourites	1.6%
Weight Watchers Chicken Suiza Enchiladas Smart Ones	1.6%
Weight Watchers Mini Rigatoni with Vodka Cream Sauce Smart Ones	1.6%
Weight Watchers Santa Fe Style Rice & Beans Smart Ones	1.6%
Weight Watchers Spicy Szechaun style vegetables & chicken Smart Ones	1.6%
Savoie's Eggs, Andouille, Potatoes & Cheese Cajun Daybreak	1.6%
El Sembrador Jamaican Style Patties Empanadas	1.6%
Jimmy Dean Bacon Skillets	1.6%
Bob Evans Original Pork Sausage & Biscuits Gravy	1.6%
Birds Eye Chicken Flavoured Rice Steamfresh	1.6%
Birds Eye Penne & Vegetables Steamfresh	1.6%
Louisa Original beef Toasted Ravioli	1.7%
Louisa Four Cheese Toasted Ravioli	1.7%
Michelina's Lasagna Alfredo	1.7%
Michelina's Fettuccine Alfredo with Chicken & Broccoli Traditional	1.7%
Farm Rich Chili Cheese Bites	1.7%
SuperPretzel Cheddar Cheese Poppers	1.7%
Lean Cuisine Chicken Alfredo Market Collection	1.7%
Stouffer's Green Pepper Steak Classics	1.7%

Frozen Dinners - by sugar content (continued)

Dinner	% sugar
Aunt Jemima Scrambled Eggs And Sausage Breakfast	1.7%
Stouffer's Grandma's Chicken & Vegetable Rice Bake Large Family	1.7%
Stouffer's Grandma's Chicken & Vegetable Rice Bake	1.7%
Stouffer's Grandma's Chicken & Vegetable Rice Bake Satisfying Servings	1.7%
Stouffer's Chicken Alfredo Skillet	1.7%
Stouffer's Grilled Chicken & Vegetables Skillet	1.7%
Stouffer's Fiesta Bake Large Family	1.7%
Innovasian Vegetable Fried Rice Family Style Side Dish	1.7%
Lean Cuisine Chicken Marsala Culinary Collection	1.7%
Stouffer's Vegetable Lasagna Farmer's Harvest	1.7%
Amy's Verde Enchilada	1.8%
Banquet Macaroni & cheese	1.8%
Michelina's Pasta With Chicken, Peas & Carrot	1.8%
Michelina's Penne with White Chicken	1.8%
Michelina's Three cheese tortellini alfredo	1.8%
Michelina's Sundried Tomato Chicken Lean Gourmet	1.8%
Michelina's Tuscan-Inspired Garlic Chicken Traditional	1.8%
Bertolli Chicken Margarita & Penne Classic meal for 7	1.8%
Bertolli Ricotta & Libster Ravioli Classic meal for 9	1.8%
Bertolli Roasted Chicken Linguine Complete Skillet meal for 2	1.8%
Bertolli Ricotta & Mozzarella Ravioli Rustico Bakes	1.8%
Stouffer's Cheesy Spaghetti Bake Classics	1.8%
Stouffer's Yankee Pot Roast Skillet	1.8%
Tai Pei Garlic Chicken	1.8%

Frozen Dinners - by sugar content (continued)

Dinner	% sugar
Stouffer's Meatloaf Satisfying Servings	1.8%
Lean Cuisine Shrimp & angel hair pasta Culinary Collection	1.8%
Lean Cuisine Macaroni & Cheese Simple Favourites	1.8%
Albuquerque Tortilla Co. Chicken With Green Chile Tamales	1.8%
Treasures from the Sea Tortilla Ranch Swai Fillet	1.8%
Banquet Spaghetti and meatballs	1.8%
Stouffer's Macaroni & Cheese Simple Dishes	1.8%
Farm Rich Breaded Mozzarella Sticks	1.8%
Gia Russa Cheese Cavatelli	1.8%
Stouffer's Salisbury Steak Classics	1.8%
Amy's Vegetable Lasagna	1.9%
Stouffer's Meat Lovers Lasagna Family	1.9%
Marie Callender's Old Fashioned Beef pot roast	1.9%
Lean Cuisine Meatloaf with Mashed Potatoes Culinary Collection	1.9%
Stouffer's Salisbury Steak	1.9%
Amy's Brown Rice, Black-Eyed Peas And Veggies Bowl	2.0%
Weight Watchers Pasta with Ricotta and Spinach Smart Ones	2.0%
Weight Watchers Shrimp Marinara Smart Ones	2.0%
Marie Callender's Chicken Corn Chowder Pot Pie	2.0%
Marie Callender's Creamy Mushroom Chicken Pot Pie	2.0%
Marie Callender's Creamy Parmesan Chicken Pot Pie	2.0%
Marie Callender's Beef pot pie	2.0%
Aunt Jemima Scrambled Eggs And Bacon Breakfast	2.0%
Marie Callender's Rigatoni Marinara Classico Pasta al dente	2.0%

Frozen Dinners - by sugar content (continued)

Dinner	% sugar
Marie Callender's Three Meat and Four Cheese Lasagna Comfort Bakes	2.0%
Banquet Cheesy beef and macaroni	2.0%
Banquet Cheesy rice and chicken	2.0%
Banquet Queso Mac	2.0%
Banquet Spaghetti and popcorn chicken	2.0%
Earth's Best Elmo Mac 'n Cheese with Carrots and Broccoli Sesame Street	2.0%
Stouffer's Lasagna with Meat & Sauce Classics	2.0%
Zatarain Shrimp Scampi with Pasta	2.0%
Lean Cuisine Baked Chicken Culinary Collection	2.0%
Michelina's Fettucine Alfredo	2.1%
Lean Cuisine Roasted Red Pepper Chicken Honestly Good	2.1%
Mrs Paul's Crunchy Fish Sticks	2.1%
Stouffer's Chicken Alfredo Large Family	2.1%
Koch Foods Broccoli & Cheese Stuffed Chicken Breast Oven Cravers	2.1%
Michelina's Pizza snack rolls	2.1%
Tai Pei Garlic Shrimp	2.1%
Stouffer's Chicken & Broccoli Pasta Bake Family	2.1%
Marie Callender's Chicken Pot Pie	2.1%
Stouffer's Creamy Chicken & Dumplings Satisfying Servings	2.1%
Green Giant Buttery Rice & Vegetables Steamers	2.1%
Stouffer's Meatloaf Classics	2.1%
Lean Cuisine Rosemary Chicken Spa Collection	2.1%
Stouffer's Cheeseburger Bake Large Family	2.1%

Frozen Dinners - by sugar content (continued)

Dinner	% sugar
Boston Market Swedish meatballs Homestyle Meals	2.2%
Banquet Chicken pasta marinara	2.2%
Birds Eye Rotini & Vegetables Steamfresh	2.2%
Amy's Black Bean & Cheese Enchilada	2.2%
Banquet Homestyle grilled meat patty	2.2%
Banquet Rigatoni with Italian sausage	2.2%
Banquet Chicken sesame	2.2%
Marie Callender's Lasagna with Meat And Sauce	2.2%
Marie Callender's Three Meat & Four Cheese Lasagna	2.2%
Michael Angelo's Chicken Parmesan	2.2%
Michelina's Spinach & ricotta bake Lean Gourmet	2.2%
Tai Pei Combination Fried rice	2.2%
Great Value Mexican Style Lasagna	2.2%
Great Value Southwest style chicken & pasta	2.2%
Lean Cuisine Stuffed cabbage Simple Favourites	2.2%
Weight Watchers Chicken Parmesan Smart Ones	2.3%
Bertolli Pappardelle Bolognese Classic meal for 8	2.4%
Contessa Tacos Fish	2.4%
Contessa Tacquitos Fish	2.4%
Hungry Man Grilled beef patty Pub Favourites	2.4%
Lean Cuisine Makhani Chicken Culinary Collection	2.4%
Morning Star Farms Veggie Buffalo Wings	2.4%
Newman's Own Chicken & Farfalle Complete Skillet Meal for Two	2.4%
Stouffer's Tuna Noodle Casserole Classics	2.4%

Frozen Dinners - by sugar content (continued)

Dinner	% sugar
Weight Watchers Chicken Santa Fe Smart Ones	2.4%
Zatarain Shrimp Alfredo	2.4%
Lean Cuisine Buffalo-Style Chicken Wrap Additions	2.4%
Marie Callender's Baked ziti marinara	2.4%
Celeste Cheesy Garlic Breadsticks	2.4%
Stouffer's Creamed Chipped Beef Classics	2.4%
Lean Cuisine Turkey Ranch Wrap Additions	2.4%
Lean Cuisine Greek-Style Chicken Salad Additions	2.4%
Marie Callender's Three Cheese Filled Rigatoni & Chicken	2.4%
Red Baron Supreme Pizza Singles	2.5%
Tai Pei Pork Potstickers	2.5%
Amy's Brown Rice & Vegetables Bowl	2.5%
Herdez Chicken Mole Bowl Cocina Mexicana	2.5%
Lean Cuisine Five Cheese Rigatoni Simple Favourites	2.5%
Marie Callender's Tortellini Romano Pasta al dente	2.5%
Stouffer's Savory Meatballs & Penne Pasta Satisfying Servings	2.5%
Lean Cuisine Chicken with Basil Cream Sauce Culinary Collection	2.5%
Michelina's Lasagna with Meat Sauce	2.5%
Healthy Choice Italian Sausage Pasta Bake Baked	2.5%
Stouffer's Chicken Lasagna Party Size	2.5%
Banquet Cheesy smothered charbroiled patties	2.5%
Green Giant Pasta, Carrots, Broccoli, Sugar Snap Peas & Garlic Sauce Steamers	2.6%
Bertolli Chicken Parmagiana & Penne Rustico Bakes	2.6%
Pagoda Express Pork Potstickers	2.6%

Frozen Dinners - by sugar content (continued)

Dinner	% sugar
Pagoda Express Chicken Potstickers	2.6%
Amy's Vegetable Korma Indian	2.6%
Stouffer's Spinach Souffle Simple Dishes	2.6%
Boston Market Spaghetti & meatballs Homestyle Meals	2.6%
Birds Eye Buffalo Style Chicken Voila	2.6%
Amy's Spinach Lasagna	2.6%
Marie Callender's Chicken, spinach & mushroom lasagna	2.6%
Michael Angelo's Meat Lasagna	2.6%
Michelina's Cheesy Chicken Ranch Lean Gourmet	2.6%
Michelina's Five cheese lasagna Lean Gourmet	2.6%
Birds Eye Cheesy Ranch Chicken Voila	2.6%
Bertolli Tuscan-Style Braised Beef With Gold Potatoes Complete Skillet meal for 3	2.6%
Stouffer's Cheesy Meatball Rigatoni Skillet	2.6%
Lean Cuisine Tortilla Crusted Fish Culinary Collection	2.7%
Patak's Chicken Tikka Masala	2.7%
Boston Market Chicken Parmesan Homestyle Meals	2.7%
Green Giant Cheesy Rice & Broccoli Steamers	2.7%
Lean Cuisine Santa Fe-Style Rice & Beans Simple Favourites	2.7%
Stouffer's Baked Ziti Large Family	2.7%
Hungry Man Mexican Style Fiesta	2.7%
Birds Eye Vegetables & shells in garlic butter sauce	2.7%
Lean Cuisine Beef pot roast Culinary Collection	2.7%
Weight Watchers Angel Hair Marinara Smart Ones	2.7%
Weight Watchers Tuna Noodle Gratin Smart Ones	2.7%

Frozen Dinners - by sugar content (continued)

Dinner	% sugar
Weight Watchers Homestyle Turkey Breast with Stuffing Smart Ones	2.7%
Boston Market Sausage & Cheese Ziti Homestyle Meals	2.8%
Banquet Zesty marinara sauce meatballs	2.8%
Healthy Choice Oven roasted chicken Complete Meals	2.8%
Tai Pei Chicken Wonton Bites	2.8%
Birds Eye Southwestern Homemade Inspirations	2.8%
Great Value Italian-Style Lasagna with Meat Sauce	2.8%
Morning Star Farms Buffalo Chik Veggie patties	2.8%
Tai Pei Chicken egg rolls	2.8%
Stouffer's Teriyaki Chicken Skillet	2.8%
Herdez Pork Chile Verde Bowl Cocina Mexicana	2.8%
Marie Callender's Chicken Alfredo	2.9%
Lean Cuisine Glazed Chicken Culinary Collection	2.9%
Bertolli Italian Sausage & Meatbal Rigatoni Rustico Bakes	2.9%
Banquet Three cheese ziti	2.9%
Weight Watchers Vegetable Fried Rice Smart Ones	2.9%
Bertolli Mushroom Lasagna Al Forno Oven bake meals	2.9%
Bertolli Manicotti Alla Vodka Rustico Bakes	2.9%
Bertolli Ziti Alforno Rustico Bakes	2.9%
Innovasian Chicken Fried Rice Family Style Side Dish	2.9%
Stouffer's Chicken Parmigiana Classics	2.9%
Stouffer's Cordon Bleu Pasta	3.0%
Lean Cuisine Southwest style chicken Salad Additions	3.0%
Morning Star Farms Tomato & Basil Pizza Veggie burgers	3.0%

Frozen Dinners - alphabetical

Brand	Dinner	% Sugar
Albie's	Albie's Chicken Pasties	0.0%
	Albie's Beef Pasties	1.5%
Albuquerque Tortilla Co.	Albuquerque Tortilla Co. Chicken With Green Chile Tamales	1.8%
Amy's	Amy's Vegetable Pie	1.4%
	Amy's Black Bean Vegetable Enchilada	1.5%
	Amy's Tofu Scramble Entrée	1.6%
	Amy's Verde Enchilada	1.8%
	Amy's Vegetable Lasagna	1.9%
	Amy's Brown Rice, Black-Eyed Peas And Veggies Bowl	2.0%
	Amy's Black Bean & Cheese Enchilada	2.2%
	Amy's Brown Rice & Vegetables Bowl	2.5%
	Amy's Vegetable Korma Indian	2.6%
	Amy's Spinach Lasagna	2.6%
An-Joy	An-Joy Chicken Fried Rice	0.4%
Atkins	Atkins Chicken & Broccoli Alfredo	0.4%
	Atkins Crustless Chicken Pot Pie	0.8%
	Atkins Meatloaf With Portebello Mushroom Gravy	0.8%
	Atkins Shrimp Scampi	0.8%
	Atkins Swedish Meatballs	0.8%
	Atkins Beef Merlot	1.2%
	Atkins Chicken Marsala	1.2%
	Atkins Italian Sausage Primavera	1.2%

Frozen Dinners - alphabetical (continued)

Brand	Dinner	% Sugar
Atkins	Atkins Orange Chicken	1.2%
	Atkins Roast Turkey Tenders With Herb Pan Gravy	1.2%
	Atkins Sesame Chicken Stir-Fry	1.2%
	Atkins Italian Style Pasta Bake	1.6%
	Atkins Mexican Style Chicken And Vegetables	1.6%
Aunt Jemima	Aunt Jemima Scrambled Eggs And Sausage Breakfast	1.7%
	Aunt Jemima Scrambled Eggs And Bacon Breakfast	2.0%
Banquet	Banquet Southwestern style patty	0.4%
	Banquet Creamy Sauce With Broccoli & Chicken Over Rice Family size	0.5%
	Banquet Fettucine Alfredo	0.5%
	Banquet Chicken nuggets and fries	0.7%
	Banquet 6 Salisbury steaks & brown gravy	0.8%
	Banquet Salisbury Steak In Gravy With Potatoes And Vegetables Family size	0.9%
	Banquet Pepper steak	0.9%
	Banquet Loaded Potato Bites	1.2%
	Banquet Mac & Cheese Bites	1.2%
	Banquet Zesty smothered meat patty	1.2%
	Banquet Chicken and broccoli pot pie	1.5%
	Banquet Macaroni & cheese	1.8%
	Banquet Spaghetti and meatballs	1.8%
	Banquet Cheesy beef and macaroni	2.0%
	Banquet Cheesy rice and chicken	2.0%

Frozen Dinners - alphabetical (continued)

Brand	Dinner	% Sugar
Banquet	Banquet Queso Mac	2.0%
	Banquet Spaghetti and popcorn chicken	2.0%
	Banquet Chicken pasta marinara	2.2%
	Banquet Homestyle grilled meat patty	2.2%
	Banquet Rigatoni with Italian sausage	2.2%
	Banquet Chicken sesame	2.2%
	Banquet Zesty marinara sauce meatballs	2.8%
	Banquet Three cheese ziti	2.9%
Barber Foods	Barber Foods Cheddar Jalepeno Stuffed chicken breasts	0.7%
	Barber Foods Loaded Baked Potato Stuffed chicken breasts	0.7%
	Barber Foods Pot Pie Taste Stuffed chicken breasts	0.7%
	Barber Foods Broccoli & Cheese Stuffed chicken breasts	0.7%
	Barber Foods Long Grain And Wild Rice Premium Entrees	1.2%
Barefoot Contessa	Barefoot Contessa Jambalaya	0.6%
	Barefoot Contessa Beef stew Bourgignon	1.3%
	Barefoot Contessa Pasta carbonara with pancetta	1.3%
	Barefoot Contessa Tequila lime chicken	1.3%
Bertolli	Bertolli Steak Rigatoni & Portabello Mushrooms Mediterranean style	0.6%
	Bertolli Chicken Florentine & Farfalle Classic meal for 4	0.9%

Frozen Dinners - alphabetical (continued)

Brand	Dinner	% Sugar
Bertolli	Bertolli Garlic Shrimp Risotto Classic meal for 2	1.2%
	Bertolli Chicken Alfredo & Penne Classic meal for 3	1.2%
	Bertolli Ricotta & Spinach Cannelloni Rustico Bakes	1.5%
	Bertolli Shrimp Scampi & Linguine Classic meal for 5	1.5%
	Bertolli Shrimp, Asparagus & Penne Classic meal for 6	1.5%
	Bertolli Grilled Chicken & Roasted Vegetables Mediterranean style	1.5%
	Bertolli Chicken Portabello Ravioli Rustico Bakes	1.5%
	Bertolli Chicken Margarita & Penne Classic meal for 7	1.8%
	Bertolli Ricotta & Libster Ravioli Classic meal for 9	1.8%
	Bertolli Roasted Chicken Linguine Complete Skillet meal for 2	1.8%
	Bertolli Ricotta & Mozzarella Ravioli Rustico Bakes	1.8%
	Bertolli Pappardelle Bolognese Classic meal for 8	2.4%
	Bertolli Chicken Parmagiana & Penne Rustico Bakes	2.6%
	Bertolli Tuscan-Style Braised Beef With Gold Potatoes Complete Skillet meal for 3	2.6%
	Bertolli Italian Sausage & Meatbal Rigatoni Rustico Bakes	2.9%
	Bertolli Mushroom Lasagna Al Forno Oven bake meals	2.9%
	Bertolli Manicotti Alla Vodka Rustico Bakes	2.9%

Frozen Dinners - alphabetical (continued)

Brand	Dinner	% Sugar
Bertolli	Bertolli Ziti Alforno Rustico Bakes	2.9%
Birds Eye	Birds Eye Chicken Florentine Voila	1.4%
	Birds Eye Chicken Flavoured Rice Steamfresh	1.6%
	Birds Eye Penne & Vegetables Steamfresh	1.6%
	Birds Eye Rotini & Vegetables Steamfresh	2.2%
	Birds Eye Buffalo Style Chicken Voila	2.6%
	Birds Eye Cheesy Ranch Chicken Voila	2.6%
	Birds Eye Southwestern Homemade Inspirations	2.8%
Bob Evans	Bob Evans Original Pork Sausage & Biscuits Gravy	1.6%
Boston Market	Boston Market Beef Steak & Pasta Homestyle Meals	0.8%
	Boston Market Buffalo Style Chicken Strips with Macaroni & Cheese Homestyle Meals	0.8%
	Boston Market Chicken, Broccoli & Cheese Casserole Homestyle Meals	0.8%
	Boston Market Turkey Breast Medallions Homestyle Meals	0.8%
	Boston Market Meatloaf & Potatoes Homestyle Bowl	0.9%
	Boston Market Southwest Style Chicken With Rice Homestyle Bowl	0.9%
	Boston Market Salisbury Steak Homestyle Meals	1.0%
	Boston Market Country Fried Chicken & Potatoes Homestyle Bowl	1.2%
	Boston Market Beef Pot Roast Homestyle Meals	1.2%
	Boston Market Chicken pot pie	1.3%

Frozen Dinners - alphabetical (continued)

Brand	Dinner	% Sugar
Boston Market	Boston Market Country Fried Beef Steak Homestyle Meals	1.3%
	Boston Market Chicken Alfredo with Fettuccine & Broccoli Homestyle Meals	1.4%
	Boston Market Turkey Breast & Potatoes Homestyle Bowl	1.5%
	Boston Market Meatloaf Homestyle Meals	1.5%
	Boston Market Swedish meatballs Homestyle Meals	2.2%
	Boston Market Spaghetti & meatballs Homestyle Meals	2.6%
	Boston Market Chicken Parmesan Homestyle Meals	2.7%
	Boston Market Sausage & Cheese Ziti Homestyle Meals	2.8%
Celeste	Celeste Cheesy Garlic Breadsticks	2.4%
Chaparro's	Chaparro's Beef Tamales	0.0%
	Chaparro's Pork Tamales	0.0%
Contessa	Contessa Empanadas Fish	1.2%
	Contessa Tacos Fish	2.4%
	Contessa Tacquitos Fish	2.4%
Culinary Delights	Culinary Delights Shrimp & sauasage jambalaya Cajun Style Selections	0.8%
	Culinary Delights Shrimp Etouffee Cajun Style Selections	0.9%
	Culinary Delights Shrimp Linguini Cajun Style Selections	0.9%
	Culinary Delights Shrimp Creole Cajun Style Selections	1.2%

Frozen Dinners - alphabetical (continued)

Brand	Dinner	% Sugar
Boston Market	Culinary Delights Creole style paella Cajun Style Selections	1.3%
Don Miguel	Don Miguel Mexican Style Lasagne Gourmet	0.9%
Earth's Best	Earth's Best Elmo Mac 'n Cheese with Carrots and Broccoli Sesame Street	2.0%
El Cazo Mexicano	El Cazo Mexicano Beef Tamales	0.0%
El Charrito	El Charrito Mexican Style Enchiladas Grande	0.2%
	El Charrito Beef echiladas Meal for Two	0.3%
	El Charrito Saltillo enchilada dinner Grande	0.6%
	El Charrito Beef & Cheese Rolled Tacos	0.7%
El Sembrador	El Sembrador Jamaican Style Patties Empanadas	1.6%
Farm Rich	Farm Rich Chili Cheese Bites	1.7%
	Farm Rich Breaded Mozzarella Sticks	1.8%
Gardenburger	Gardenburger The original Veggie burgers	0.0%
Gia Russa	Gia Russa Stuffed rigatoni	1.2%
	Gia Russa Tri-Colored Tortellini	1.2%
	Gia Russa Manicotti With Ricotta Cheese	1.3%
	Gia Russa Cheese Cavatelli	1.8%
Gluten Free Café	Gluten Free Café Lemon Basil Chicken	0.8%
Great Value	Great Value Shrimp Scampi & Linguini	0.9%
	Great Value Grilled Chicken Alfredo	1.5%
	Great Value Chicken Enchilada Casserole	1.5%
	Great Value Mexican Style Lasagna	2.2%

Frozen Dinners - alphabetical (continued)

Brand	Dinner	% Sugar
Green Giant	Green Giant Cheesy Rice & Broccoli Just for One	0.8%
	Green Giant Buttery Rice & Vegetables Steamers	2.1%
Green Giant	Green Giant Pasta, Carrots, Broccoli, Sugar Snap Peas & Garlic Sauce Steamers	2.6%
	Green Giant Cheesy Rice & Broccoli Steamers	2.7%
Hanover	Hanover Caribbean Black Beans in Sauce Bean Essentials	0.0%
	Hanover Tuscan White Beans in Sauce Bean Essentials	0.8%
	Hanover Cajun Pink Beans in Sauce Bean Essentials	1.5%
	Hanover Southwestern Pinto Beans in Sauce Bean Essentials	1.5%
Healthy Choice	Healthy Choice Fettuccini Alfredo Bake Baked	0.4%
	Healthy Choice Chicken Enchilada Bake Baked	0.8%
	Healthy Choice Chicken & Rice Cheddar Bake Baked	0.8%
	Healthy Choice Chicken & Spinach Alfredo Baked	0.8%
	Healthy Choice Roasted Chicken and Potatoes Baked	1.1%
	Healthy Choice Italian Sausage Pasta Bake Baked	2.5%
	Healthy Choice Oven roasted chicken Complete Meals	2.8%
Herdez	Herdez Carnitas & Charro Beans Bowl Cocina Mexicana	0.0%
	Herdez Pork Chile Colorado Bowl Cocina Mexicana	0.4%

Frozen Dinners - alphabetical (continued)

Brand	Dinner	% Sugar
Herdez	Herdez Beef Barbacoa Bowl Cocina Mexicana	0.7%
	Herdez Chicken Chipotle Bowl Cocina Mexicana	0.7%
	Herdez Huevos Rancheros Bowl Cocina Mexicana	0.7%
	Herdez Pork al Pastor Bowl Cocina Mexicana	1.4%
	Herdez Chicken Mole Bowl Cocina Mexicana	2.5%
	Herdez Pork Chile Verde Bowl Cocina Mexicana	2.8%
Hungry Man	Hungry Man Grilled beef patty Pub Favourites	2.4%
	Hungry Man Mexican Style Fiesta	2.7%
Innovasian	Innovasian Vegetable Fried Rice Family Style Side Dish	1.7%
	Innovasian Chicken Fried Rice Family Style Side Dish	2.9%
Jimmy Dean	Jimmy Dean Bacon Breakfast Bowl	0.0%
	Jimmy Dean Sausage Breakfast Bowl	0.0%
	Jimmy Dean Sausage & gravy Breakfast bowl	0.4%
	Jimmy Dean Sausage Skillets	0.8%
	Jimmy Dean Bacon Skillets	1.6%
Koch Foods	Koch Foods Cordon Bleu Oven Cravers	1.4%
	Koch Foods Broccoli & Cheese Stuffed Chicken Breast Oven Cravers	2.1%
Lean Cuisine	Lean Cuisine Grilled Chicken Caesar Culinary Collection	0.8%
	Lean Cuisine Steak Portabello Culinary Collection	0.9%
	Lean Cuisine Lemon Pepper fish Culinary Collection	1.2%

Frozen Dinners - alphabetical (continued)

Brand	Dinner	% Sugar
Lean Cuisine	Lean Cuisine Chicken Fried Rice Simple Favourites	1.6%
	Lean Cuisine Chicken Alfredo Market Collection	1.7%
	Lean Cuisine Chicken Marsala Culinary Collection	1.7%
	Lean Cuisine Shrimp & angel hair pasta Culinary Collection	1.8%
	Lean Cuisine Macaroni & Cheese Simple Favourites	1.8%
	Lean Cuisine Meatloaf with Mashed Potatoes Culinary Collection	1.9%
	Lean Cuisine Baked Chicken Culinary Collection	2.0%
	Lean Cuisine Roasted Red Pepper Chicken Honestly Good	2.1%
	Lean Cuisine Rosemary Chicken Spa Collection	2.1%
	Lean Cuisine Stuffed cabbage Simple Favourites	2.2%
	Lean Cuisine Makhani Chicken Culinary Collection	2.4%
	Lean Cuisine Buffalo-Style Chicken Wrap Additions	2.4%
	Lean Cuisine Turkey Ranch Wrap Additions	2.4%
	Lean Cuisine Greek-Style Chicken Salad Additions	2.4%
	Lean Cuisine Five Cheese Rigatoni Simple Favourites	2.5%
	Lean Cuisine Chicken with Basil Cream Sauce Culinary Collection	2.5%
	Lean Cuisine Tortilla Crusted Fish Culinary Collection	2.7%

Frozen Dinners - alphabetical (continued)

Brand	Dinner	% Sugar
Lean Cuisine	Lean Cuisine Santa Fe-Style Rice & Beans Simple Favourites	2.7%
	Lean Cuisine Beef pot roast Culinary Collection	2.7%
	Lean Cuisine Glazed Chicken Culinary Collection	2.9%
	Lean Cuisine Southwest style chicken Salad Additions	3.0%
Louisa	Louisa Sausage & Cheese Toasted Ravioli	0.8%
	Louisa Original beef Toasted Ravioli	1.7%
	Louisa Four Cheese Toasted Ravioli	1.7%
Marie Callender's	Marie Callender's Braised Beef Pot Roast Comfort Bakes	0.0%
	Marie Callender's Savory Chicken & Rice Comfort Bakes	0.0%
	Marie Callender's Egg Cheese & Ham Bake Breakfast Anytime	0.4%
	Marie Callender's Cheesy Egg & Sausage Bake Breakfast Anytime	0.5%
	Marie Callender's Meat Loaf & Gravy	0.5%
	Marie Callender's Turkey Breast & Stuffing	0.5%
	Marie Callender's Chunky Chicken & noodles	0.5%
	Marie Callender's Penne Chicken Modesto Pasta al dente	0.6%
	Marie Callender's Country Fried Chicken & Gravy	0.7%
	Marie Callender's Cheddar & Bacon Potato Bake Comfort Bakes	0.7%
	Marie Callender's Chicken & Broccoli Alfredo Comfort Bakes	0.7%

Frozen Dinners - alphabetical (continued)

Brand	Dinner	% Sugar
Marie Callender's	Marie Callender's Cheesy Chicken & Rice Comfort Bakes	0.8%
	Marie Callender's Vermont white cheddar mac & cheese	0.9%
	Marie Callender's Creamy Chicken alfredo with sundried tomatoes	0.9%
	Marie Callender's Steak & Roasted Potatoes	1.0%
	Marie Callender's Scalloped Potatoes with Ham	1.1%
	Marie Callender's Salisbury steak	1.3%
	Marie Callender's Turkey pot pie	1.4%
	Marie Callender's Mac and Cheese	1.4%
	Marie Callender's Golden battered fish fillet	1.5%
	Marie Callender's Old Fashioned Beef pot roast	1.9%
	Marie Callender's Chicken Corn Chowder Pot Pie	2.0%
	Marie Callender's Creamy Mushroom Chicken Pot Pie	2.0%
	Marie Callender's Creamy Parmesan Chicken Pot Pie	2.0%
	Marie Callender's Beef pot pie	2.0%
	Marie Callender's Rigatoni Marinara Classico Pasta al dente	2.0%
	Marie Callender's Three Meat and Four Cheese Lasagna Comfort Bakes	2.0%
	Marie Callender's Chicken Pot Pie	2.1%
	Marie Callender's Lasagna with Meat And Sauce	2.2%

Frozen Dinners - alphabetical (continued)

Brand	Dinner	% Sugar
Marie Callender's	Marie Callender's Three Meat & Four Cheese Lasagna	2.2%
	Marie Callender's Baked ziti marinara	2.4%
	Marie Callender's Three Cheese Filled Rigatoni & Chicken	2.4%
	Marie Callender's Tortellini Romano Pasta al dente	2.5%
	Marie Callender's Chicken, spinach & mushroom lasagna	2.6%
	Marie Callender's Chicken Alfredo	2.9%
McKenzie's	McKenzie's Southern Field Peas With Snaps	0.0%
Michael Angelo's	Michael Angelo's Chicken Piccata	0.7%
	Michael Angelo's Chicken Parmesan	2.2%
	Michael Angelo's Meat Lasagna	2.6%
Michelina's	Michelina's Salisbury Steak Traditional	0.4%
	Michelina's Pop'n Chicken Traditional	0.7%
	Michelina's Sante Fe style rice & beans Lean Gourmet	0.8%
	Michelina's Macaroni & cheese	0.9%
	Michelina's Sante Fe style rice & beans	0.9%
	Michelina's Wheels & Cheese Pasta	0.9%
	Michelina's Buffalo-Style Chicken Mac & Cheese	0.9%
	Michelina's Broccoli Cheese Chicken Lean Gourmet	0.9%
	Michelina's Chicken Asiago Lean Gourmet	0.9%
	Michelina's Creamy rigatoni with broccoli & chicken Lean Gourmet	0.9%

Frozen Dinners - alphabetical (continued)

Brand	Dinner	% Sugar
Michelina's	Michelina's Three cheese chicken Lean Gourmet	0.9%
	Michelina's Stir fry rice & vegetables with chicken Lean Gourmet	0.9%
	Michelina's Chicken Fried Rice Traditional	0.9%
	Michelina's Cheeseburger Mac	1.3%
	Michelina's Chicken alfredo florentine Lean Gourmet	1.3%
	Michelina's Chipotle Chicken & Rice Lean Gourmet	1.3%
	Michelina's Beef & Peppers Traditional	1.3%
	Michelina's White Turkey in Cream Sauce with Pasta Traditional	1.3%
	Michelina's Meatloaf Lean Gourmet	1.4%
	Michelina's Lasagna Alfredo	1.7%
	Michelina's Fettuccine Alfredo with Chicken & Broccoli Traditional	1.7%
	Michelina's Pasta With Chicken, Peas & Carrot	1.7%
	Michelina's Penne with White Chicken	1.8%
	Michelina's Three cheese tortellini alfredo	1.8%
	Michelina's Sundried Tomato Chicken Lean Gourmet	1.8%
	Michelina's Tuscan-Inspired Garlic Chicken Traditional	1.8%
	Michelina's Fettucine Alfredo	2.1%
	Michelina's Pizza snack rolls	2.1%
	Michelina's Spinach & ricotta bake Lean Gourmet	2.2%
	Michelina's Lasagna with Meat Sauce	2.5%

Frozen Dinners - alphabetical (continued)

Brand	Dinner	% Sugar
Michelina's	Michelina's Cheesy Chicken Ranch Lean Gourmet	2.6%
	Michelina's Five cheese lasagna Lean Gourmet	2.6%
Morning Star Farms	Morning Star Farms Mushroom Lover's Veggie burgers	0.0%
	Morning Star Farms Veggie meatballs	1.3%
	Morning Star Farms original Chik Veggie patties	1.4%
	Morning Star Farms Mediterranean Chickpea Veggie burgers	1.5%
	Morning Star Farms Roasted Garlic & Quinoa Veggie burgers	1.5%
	Morning Star Farms Spicy Black Bean Veggie burgers	1.5%
	Morning Star Farms California Turk'y Grillers	1.6%
	Morning Star Farms Veggie Buffalo Wings	2.4%
	Morning Star Farms Buffalo Chik Veggie patties	2.8%
	Morning Star Farms Tomato & Basil Pizza Veggie burgers	3.0%
Mrs Paul's	Mrs Paul's Crunchy Fish Sticks	2.1%
Mrs T's	Mrs T's Potato & onion Pierogies	0.9%
	Mrs T's Potato & onion mini Pierogies	1.2%
Newman's Own	Newman's Own Chicken Florentine & Farfalle Complete Skillet Meal for Two	1.2%
	Newman's Own Chicken Parmigiana & Penne Complete Skillet Meal for Two	1.2%
	Newman's Own Italian Sausage & Rigatoni Complete Skillet Meal for Two	1.2%
	Newman's Own Chicken & Farfalle Complete Skillet Meal for Two	2.4%

Frozen Dinners - alphabetical (continued)

Brand	Dinner	% Sugar
Night Hawk	Night Hawk Charbroiled bites & Taters	0.0%
	Night Hawk Steak 'N Taters	0.0%
	Night Hawk Top Chop't Classic	0.9%
	Night Hawk Beef Patty 'N Gravy	1.2%
	Night Hawk Beef Patty 'N Mashed Potatoes	1.4%
	Night Hawk Taste of texas	1.5%
On-Cor	On-Cor Chicken Fettucine Alfredo	1.1%
Ore-Ida	Ore-Ida Shredded Hash Brown Potatoes	1.1%
	Ore-Ida Tater Tots	1.2%
	Ore-Ida Potatoes O'Brien with Onions & Peppers	1.2%
	Ore-Ida Seasoned Crinkles Extra Crispy	1.2%
	Ore-Ida Fast Food Fries Extra Crispy	1.2%
	Ore-Ida Golden Crinkles Extra Crispy	1.2%
	Ore-Ida Golden fries	1.2%
	Ore-Ida Shoestrings	1.2%
	Ore-Ida Waffle Fries	1.2%
Ore-Ida	Ore-Ida Zesties	1.2%
	Ore-Ida Zesty Twirls	1.2%
Owens	Owens Sausage Biscuits Snackwiches	0.0%
	Owens Sausage Egg & Cheese Tacos Border Breakfasts	1.5%
Pagoda Express	Pagoda Express Chicken Fried Rice	0.6%
	Pagoda Express Pork Potstickers	2.6%
	Pagoda Express Chicken Potstickers	2.6%

Frozen Dinners - alphabetical (continued)

Brand	Dinner	% Sugar
Patak's	Patak's Chicken Tikka Masala	2.7%
Quirch Foods	Quirch Foods Jerk Chicken Jamaican Style Patties	0.8%
Red Baron	Red Baron Supreme Pizza Singles	2.5%
Rice Gourmet	Rice Gourmet Chicken Fried Rice	1.1%
Richard's Cajun Favourites	Richard's Cajun Favourites Seafood Jambalaya	0.6%
	Richard's Cajun Favourites Shrimp Etouffee	0.6%
	Richard's Cajun Favourites Crawfish Etouffee	1.0%
	Richard's Cajun Favourites Chicken Fettucine	1.2%
	Richard's Cajun Favourites Pork & Sausage Jambalaya	1.2%
Savoie's	Savoie's Eggs, Andouille & Potatoes with Gravy Cajun Daybreak	0.5%
	Savoie's Chicken & Sausage Jambalaya Cajun Singles	0.7%
	Savoie's Eggs, Andouille, Potatoes & Cheese Cajun Daybreak	1.6%
Snapps	Snapps Cheese Sticks Snackbites	0.0%
	Snapps Loaded potato sticks Snackbites	1.1%
	Snapps Cheeseburger Fritters	1.3%
Southern Belle	Southern Belle Lobster Mac-N-Cheese	0.8%
Stouffer's	Stouffer's Escalloped Chicken & Noodles Classics	0.6%
	Stouffer's Braised Beef & Roasted Red Skin Potatoes Satisfying Servings	0.7%
	Stouffer's Fish Fillet Classics	0.8%

Frozen Dinners - alphabetical (continued)

Brand	Dinner	% Sugar
Stouffer's	Stouffer's Escalloped Chicken & Noodles Family	0.8%
	Stouffer's Rigatoni Pasta with Roasted White Meat Chicken Classics	0.8%
	Stouffer's Savory Chicken & Rice Skillet	0.9%
	Stouffer's Roast Turkey Breast Satisfying Servings	0.9%
	Stouffer's Roast Turkey Classics	1.1%
	Stouffer's Broccoli & Beef Skillet Easy Express	1.1%
	Stouffer's Macaroni & Cheese Broccoli Classics	1.2%
	Stouffer's Chicken Fettuccini Alfredo Satisfying Servings	1.2%
	Stouffer's Braised beef & portebello tortellini Sautes for Two	1.2%
	Stouffer's Baked Chicken Breast Classics	1.2%
	Stouffer's Beef Pot Roast Classics	1.2%
	Stouffer's Cheesy Chicken & Broccoli Rice Bake	1.2%
	Stouffer's Grilled Chicken & Asiago Tortellini Sautes for Two	1.2%
	Stouffer's Chicken a la King Classics	1.2%
	Stouffer's Savory Beef & Vegetables Satisfying Servings	1.3%
	Stouffer's Garlic shrimp skillet Easy Express	1.3%
	Stouffer's Meatloaf	1.3%
	Stouffer's Salisbury Steak Satisfying Servings	1.3%
	Stouffer's Homestyle Beef Skillet	1.4%
	Stouffer's Grilled Asiago Chicken & Penne Pasta Satisfying Servings	1.4%

Frozen Dinners - alphabetical (continued)

Brand	Dinner	% Sugar
Stouffer's	Stouffer's Rigatoni with Chicken & Pesto Family	1.4%
	Stouffer's Turkey Tetrazzini Classics	1.5%
	Stouffer's Chicken & Dumplings Skillet	1.5%
	Stouffer's Savory Beef & Vegetables	1.5%
	Stouffer's Swedish Meatballs Classics	1.5%
	Stouffer's Green Pepper Steak Classics	1.7%
	Stouffer's Grandma's Chicken & Vegetable Rice Bake Large Family	1.7%
	Stouffer's Grandma's Chicken & Vegetable Rice Bake	1.7%
	Stouffer's Grandma's Chicken & Vegetable Rice Bake Satisfying Servings	1.7%
	Stouffer's Chicken Alfredo Skillet	1.7%
	Stouffer's Grilled Chicken & Vegetables Skillet	1.7%
	Stouffer's Fiesta Bake Large Family	1.7%
	Stouffer's Vegetable Lasagna Farmer's Harvest	1.7%
	Stouffer's Cheesy Spaghetti Bake Classics	1.8%
	Stouffer's Yankee Pot Roast Skillet	1.8%
	Stouffer's Meatloaf Satisfying Servings	1.8%
	Stouffer's Macaroni & Cheese Simple Dishes	1.8%
	Stouffer's Salisbury Steak Classics	1.8%
	Stouffer's Meat Lovers Lasagna Family	1.9%
	Stouffer's Salisbury Steak	1.9%
	Stouffer's Lasagna with Meat & Sauce Classics	2.0%
	Stouffer's Chicken Alfredo Large Family	2.1%

Frozen Dinners - alphabetical (continued)

Brand	Dinner	% Sugar
Stouffer's	Stouffer's Chicken & Broccoli Pasta Bake Family	2.1%
	Stouffer's Creamy Chicken & Dumplings Satisfying Servings	2.1%
	Stouffer's Meatloaf Classics	2.1%
	Stouffer's Cheeseburger Bake Large Family	2.1%
	Stouffer's Tuna Noodle Casserole Classics	2.4%
	Stouffer's Creamed Chipped Beef Classics	2.4%
	Stouffer's Savory Meatballs & Penne Pasta Satisfying Servings	2.5%
	Stouffer's Chicken Lasagna Party Size	2.5%
	Stouffer's Spinach Souffle Simple Dishes	2.6%
	Stouffer's Cheesy Meatball Rigatoni Skillet	2.6%
	Stouffer's Baked Ziti Large Family	2.7%
Stouffer's	Stouffer's Teriyaki Chicken Skillet	2.8%
	Stouffer's Chicken Parmigiana Classics	2.9%
	Stouffer's Cordon Bleu Pasta	3.0%
SuperPretzel	SuperPretzel Cheddar Cheese Poppers	1.7%
T.G.I. Friday's	T.G.I. Friday's Buffalo Style Sauce Boneless Chicken Bites	0.0%
	T.G.I. Friday's Cheddar & Bacon Potato Skins	1.0%
	T.G.I. Friday's Cheese & Bacon Loaded Fries	1.2%
Tai Pei	Tai Pei Chicken fried rice	0.6%
	Tai Pei Shrimp Fried rice	1.4%
	Tai Pei Chicken Chow Mein	1.5%
	Tai Pei Garlic Chicken	1.8%

Frozen Dinners - alphabetical (continued)

Brand	Dinner	% Sugar
Tai Pei	Tai Pei Garlic Shrimp	2.1%
	Tai Pei Combination Fried rice	2.2%
	Tai Pei Pork Potstickers	2.5%
	Tai Pei Chicken Wonton Bites	2.8%
	Tai Pei Chicken egg rolls	2.8%
Treasures from the Sea	Treasures from the Sea Butter Herb Shrimp	0.9%
	Treasures from the Sea Tortilla Ranch Swai Fillet	1.8%
Weight Watchers	Weight Watchers Chicken Strips & Fries Smart Ones	0.0%
	Weight Watchers Slow Roasted Turkey Breast Smart Ones	0.0%
	Weight Watchers Ham and Cheese Scramble Smart Ones	0.5%
	Weight Watchers Chicken Fettuccini Smart Ones	0.8%
	Weight Watchers Creamy Rigatoni with Broccoli & Chicken Smart Ones	0.8%
	Weight Watchers Meatloaf Smart Ones	0.8%
	Weight Watchers Roast Beef, Mashed Potatoes and Gravy Smart Ones	0.8%
	Weight Watchers Salisbury Steak Smart Ones	0.8%
	Weight Watchers Salisbury Steak Smart Ones	1.1%
	Weight Watchers Chicken Oriental Smart Ones	1.2%
	Weight Watchers Three Cheese Ziti Marinara Smart Ones	1.2%
	Weight Watchers Beef Pot Roast Smart Ones	1.2%

Frozen Dinners - alphabetical (continued)

Brand	Dinner	% Sugar
Weight Watchers	Weight Watchers Chicken Fajitas Smart Ones	1.3%
	Weight Watchers Steak Fajitas Smart Ones	1.3%
	Weight Watchers Chicken Suiza Enchiladas Smart Ones	1.6%
	Weight Watchers Mini Rigatoni with Vodka Cream Sauce Smart Ones	1.6%
	Weight Watchers Santa Fe Style Rice & Beans Smart Ones	1.6%
	Weight Watchers Spicy Szechaun style vegetables & chicken Smart Ones	1.6%
	Weight Watchers Pasta with Ricotta and Spinach Smart Ones	2.0%
	Weight Watchers Shrimp Marinara Smart Ones	2.0%
	Weight Watchers Chicken Parmesan Smart Ones	2.3%
	Weight Watchers Chicken Santa Fe Smart Ones	2.4%
	Weight Watchers Angel Hair Marinara Smart Ones	2.7%
	Weight Watchers Tuna Noodle Gratin Smart Ones	2.7%
	Weight Watchers Homestyle Turkey Breast with Stuffing Smart Ones	2.7%
	Weight Watchers Vegetable Fried Rice Smart Ones	2.9%
Zatarain	Zatarain With Beef & Pork Dirty Rice	0.4%
	Zatarain Chicken & Sausage Jambalaya Meal For Two	0.6%
	Zatarain Smothered Chicken & Rice Meal For Two	0.6%
	Zatarain Flavored With Sausage Jambalaya	0.9%

Frozen Dinners - alphabetical (continued)

Brand	Dinner	% Sugar
Zatarain	Zatarain Beef & Mushroom Pasta Meal For Two	0.9%
	Zatarain Sausage & Chicken Gumbo With Rice	0.9%
	Zatarain With Yellow Rice Blackened Chicken	1.0%
	Zatarain With Sausage Red Beans & Rice	1.5%
	Zatarain Shrimp Scampi with Pasta	2.0%
	Zatarain Shrimp Alfredo	2.4%

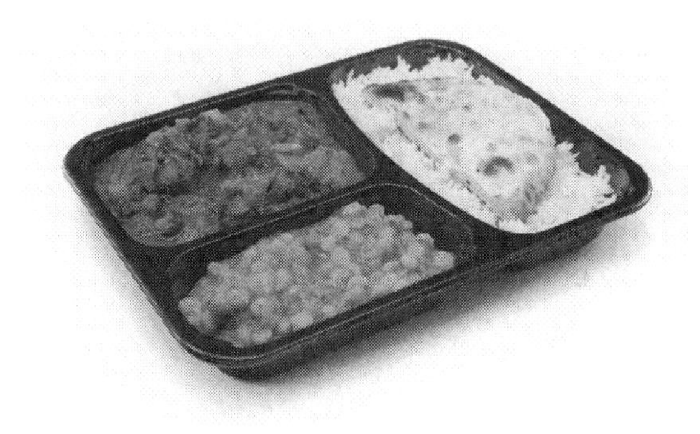

Boxed Meals

I've presented this list in two formats so you can browse by sugar content or brand.

Most of these boxed meals will contain seed oils. If you are concerned about this, then use the fat reckoner chart available at www.howmuchsugar.com to determine whether your choice is likely to be as low in seed oil as it is in sugar.

Boxed Meals - by sugar content

Meal	% Sugar
Betty Crocker Creamy Butter Mashed Potatoes	0.0%
Betty Crocker Riasted Garlic Mashed Potatoes	0.0%
Betty Crocker Scalloped Potatoes	0.0%
Conchita Extra Fancy Long Grain Rice	0.0%
Conchita Long Grain Brown Rice	0.0%
Conchita Parboiled Long Grain Rice	0.0%
Fiesta Round Duros	0.0%
Gillian's Wheat and gluten free Home-style Stuffing	0.0%
Gourmantra Tandoori Indian Meal Kit	0.0%
Great Value Au Gratin Potatoes	0.0%
Great Value Creamy Butter Instant Mashed Potatoes	0.0%
Great Value Mashed Potatoes	0.0%
Hormel Smoky bacon parmesan rigatoni Compleats	0.0%
Hormel Chicken Breast & mashed potato Compleats Homestyle	0.0%
Hungry Jack Naturally flavoured Mashed Potatoes	0.0%
Kitchens of India Rajma Masala red kidney beans Curry	0.0%

Boxed Meals - by sugar content (continued)

Meal	% Sugar
Knorr Buffalo chicken rice Rice sides	0.0%
Kohinoor Punjabi kadhi pakora	0.0%
Kartoffelland Raw potato dumplings	0.0%
La Tiara Mexican taco shells	0.0%
Louisiana Cajun Etouffee Mix	0.0%
Louisiana Cajun Gumbo mix	0.0%
Louisiana Seasoned chicken fry	0.0%
Luzianne Jambalaya dinner kit	0.0%
Marcy's Traditional stuffing mix	0.0%
McCormick Paella Rice	0.0%
Rice-a-Roni Rice pilaf	0.0%
St Dalfour Tuna & pasta Gourmet on the go	0.0%
St Dalfour Wild salmon with vegetables Gourmet on the go	0.0%
St Dalfour Three beans with sweetcorn Gourmet on the go	0.0%
TGI Fridays Buffalo style sauce Chicken wings	0.0%
Thai Kitchen Stir-fry rice noodles	0.0%
Truly Indian Chatpate Choley	0.0%
Truly Indian Matar paneer	0.0%
Zatarain's Dirty Big Easy rice	0.0%
Zatarain's Jambalaya Big Easy rice	0.0%
Zatarain's Red rice & beans Big Easy rice	0.0%
Zatarain's Gumbo mix	0.0%
Zatarain's Dirty brown rice New Orleans Style	0.0%
Zatarain's Etouffee base New Orleans Style	0.0%
Zatarain's Original dirty rice New Orleans Style	0.0%

Boxed Meals - by sugar content (continued)

Meal	% Sugar
Zatarain's Original Jambalaya rice New Orleans Style	0.0%
Ziyad Roasted Green wheat Pilaf	0.0%
Ziyad Rice & lentil Pilaf	0.0%
Kohinoor Dal palak with rice & curry	0.3%
Hormel Italian herb & cheese rigatoni Compleats	0.4%
Hormel Roast beef & gravy with mashed potatoes Compleats	0.4%
Hormel Salisbury steak with sliced potatoes & gravy Compleats	0.4%
Hormel Macaroni & cheese Compleats Homestyle	0.4%
Patak's Potato & spinach curry	0.4%
Hormel Three cheese chicken pasta Compleats	0.4%
Hormel Bacon breakfast scramble Compleats Good Mornings	0.5%
Betty Crocker Chicken with Cheesy Rice & Broccoli Helper Complete Meals	0.6%
Tasty Bite Kashmir spinach	0.7%
Hormel Chicken & rice Compleats	0.7%
Nalley Beef in chilli sauce Tamales	0.7%
Sam Miguel White rice with vegetables	0.7%
Kitchens of India Chickpea Curry	0.8%
Kitchens of India Spinach palak paneer Curry	0.8%
Taste of Bombay Chicken Tikka Masala	0.8%
Kohinoor Madras lemon rice with sambhar	0.9%
Jyoti with spinach Mung dal	0.9%
Hormel Sausage breakfast scramble Compleats Good Mornings	0.9%
Udon Mushroom Noodles	1.0%

Boxed Meals - by sugar content (continued)

Meal	% Sugar
Patel's Potato & Green pea Curry	1.0%
TruRoots Curry rice multigrain Pilaf	1.0%
La Choy Asian fried rice Creations	1.0%
Banquet Cheesy Ham & Hash Brown Homestyle Bakes	1.0%
Dinty Moore Beef Stew	1.1%
Hormel Chicken & Dumplings Microwave Bowls	1.1%
Hormel Beef Pot Roast Compleats Homestyle	1.1%
Hormel Chicken Breast & Dressing Compleats Homestyle	1.1%
Hormel Meatloaf & mashed potatoes Compleats Homestyle	1.1%
Patak's Lentil curry	1.1%
Vigo Yellow rice & seafood dinner	1.1%
Hormel Creamy Cheese & Basil tortellini Compleats	1.2%
Road's End Organics Alfredo style Mac & cheese	1.2%
Road's End Organics Cheddar style Penne & Cheese	1.2%
Weight Watchers Three cheese omelette Smart Ones	1.2%
Betty Crocker Fried Rice with Chicken Helper Complete Meals	1.2%
Uncle Ben's Teriyaki Ready Rice	1.3%
Margaret Holmes Creole fixins Simple Suppers	1.3%
Patel's Basmati rice with green peas	1.4%
Hormel Sausage Gravy & roasted potatoes Compleats Good Mornings	1.4%
Hormel Cheesy diced potatoes Country Crock	1.4%
Hormel Beef Steak & Peppers Compleats	1.4%
Hormel Chicken Pasta Primavera Compleats	1.4%
Hormel Turkey & dressing with gravy Compleats	1.4%

Boxed Meals - by sugar content (continued)

Meal	% Sugar
Patak's Butter chicken with rice	1.4%
Spam Spam & cheesy potatoes Meal for 1	1.4%
Kitchens of India with vegetable & nuts Basmati rice pilaf	1.4%
Zatarain's Garden vegetable brown rice Big Easy rice	1.4%
McCormick Chicken flavour Rice	1.5%
Banquet Dumplings & Chicken Homestyle Bakes	1.6%
Healthy Choices Beef & Broccoli Modern Classics	1.6%
Cugino's Creamy Roasted Red Pepper Pasta Sides	1.6%
Knorr Steak fajitas rice Rice sides	1.6%
Banquet Creamy Turkey & Stuffing Homestyle Bakes	1.6%
Knorr Rice pilaf Rice sides	1.6%
Cugino's Mushroom Stroganoff Pasta Sides	1.7%
Knorr Chicken Pasta Sides	1.7%
Taco Bell Crunchy & soft Taco dinner kit	1.7%
Banquet Chicken, Mashed Potato and Biscuits Homestyle Bakes	1.7%
Louisiana Purchase Jambalaya rice mix	1.8%
Slap Ya Mama Cajun Jambalaya Mix	1.8%
Slap Ya Mama Cajun Red beans & rice	1.8%
Zatarain's Red beans & rice New Orleans Style	1.8%
Zatarain's Wild brown rice	1.8%
Hormel Spaghetti & turkey meatballs Compleats	1.8%
Patak's Chicken curry	1.8%
Spam Spam & roasted potatoes with gravy Meal for 2	1.8%
A Taste of Thai Coconut Ginger Noodles	1.8%
Barilla Three Cheese Tortellini	1.8%

Boxed Meals - by sugar content (continued)

Meal	% Sugar
Near East Roasted vegetable & chicken Long grain and wild rice	1.8%
Near East Toasted almond Rice pilaf mix	1.8%
Rice-a-Roni Chicken Rice & Vermicelli mix	1.8%
Rice-a-Roni Chicken teriyaki Rice & Vermicelli mix	1.8%
Vigo Long grain white & wild rice	1.8%
Vigo Seasoned risotto with broccoli	1.8%
Betty Crocker Cheesy Chicken Helper Complete Meals	1.8%
Domo Four Cheese Risotto	1.8%
Domo Mushrooms Risotto	1.8%
Old el Paso Carne Asada steak Tortilla stuffers	1.8%
Betty Crocker Cheesy Beef taco Helper Complete Meals	1.8%
Betty Crocker Chicken & Buttermilk Biscuits Helper Complete Meals	1.8%
Betty Crocker Stroganoff Helper Complete Meals	1.8%
Betty Crocker Chicken Fettuccine Alfredo Helper Complete Meals	1.8%
Birds Eye Lightly sauced roasted red potatoes and green beans Steamfresh	1.9%
Annie's Homegrown Rice Pasta & Extra Cheesy Cheddar Creamy Deluxe	1.9%
Kraft Chicken Alfredo Velveeta Cheesy Skillets	2.0%
Kraft Chicken Chilli Cheese mac Velveeta Cheesy Skillets	2.0%
Kohinoor Mutter paneer	2.0%
Old el Paso Garlic Chili chicken Tortilla stuffers	2.0%
Osem Mejadar rice & lentils	2.0%
Side Mates Original pearl couscous	2.0%

Boxed Meals - by sugar content (continued)

Meal	% Sugar
SuperPretzel Cheese filled Softstix	2.0%
Tasty Bite Aloo Palak	2.1%
Tasty Bite Bombay Potatoes	2.1%
Tasty Bite Jaipur Vegetables	2.1%
Tasty Bite Spinach channa	2.1%
Spam Spam & scalloped potatoes Meal for 3	2.1%
Annie's Homegrown Elbows & Four Cheese Creamy Deluxe	2.1%
Kitchens of India with vegetables Basmati rice pilaf	2.1%
Laurie's Kitchen Chicken Parmesan truffle	2.2%
Maggi Spaetzle dumplings	2.2%
Tony Chachere's Creole yellow rice	2.2%
Tony Chachere's Dirty rice Dry Creole	2.2%
Annie's Homegrown Macaroni Creamy Deluxe	2.2%
Banquet Creamy Cheesy Chicken Alfredo Homestyle Bakes	2.2%
Goya Chicken Mexican Rice	2.2%
Heritage Select Roasted Chicken and Herb Basmati	2.2%
Heritage Select Roasted Garlic and Herb Basmati	2.2%
Louisiana Dirty rice mix	2.2%
Augason Farms 72 Hour 1 person Emergency Kit	2.3%
Ready Pac Foods Bistro Chef Salad	2.3%
Nongshim Spicy Chicken Noodle soup	2.3%
Kraft Lasagna with meat Velveeta Cheesy Skillets	2.4%
Kraft Ultimate Cheeseburger Velveeta Cheesy Skillets	2.4%
Kraft Hearty Four Cheese Homestyle Macaroni & Cheese	2.4%
Mrs Leeper's Creamy tuna & pasta mix	2.4%

Boxed Meals - by sugar content (continued)

Meal	% Sugar
Osem Couscous & vegetables Meals on the go	2.4%
Kitchens of India Pav Bhaji mashed vegetable Curry	2.4%
Hamburger Helper Crunchy Taco	2.4%
Taco Bell Crunchy Taco dinner kit	2.4%
Old el Paso Stand N Stuff Taco dinner kit	2.5%
Hormel Cheese & Spinach Compleats	2.5%
Hidden Valley Original Ranch Pasta Salad	2.5%
Zatarain's Brown rice jambalaya mix New Orleans Style	2.5%
Banquet Biscuits & Chicken Homestyle Bakes	2.5%
Banquet Sausage Gravy & Biscuits Homestyle Bakes	2.5%
Healthy Choices Herb Crusted Fish Modern Classics	2.6%
Hidden Valley Southwest Ranch Pasta Salad	2.6%
Tony Chachere's Jambalaya dinner mix Dry Creole	2.6%
Jyoti with zucchini Channa dal	2.6%
Zatarain's Jambalaya pasta dinner New Orleans Style	2.6%
Zatarain's Spanish rice New Orleans Style	2.7%
Zatarain's Southern stroganoff Pasta dinner	2.7%
Barilla Marinara Penne Italian Entrees	2.7%
Sam Mills Alfredo Gluten Free Pasta Sides	2.8%
TruRoots Mediterranean vegetable multigrain Pilaf	2.8%
Tasty Bite Peas Paneer	2.8%
Tasty Bite Vegetable Korma	2.8%
Hormel Chilli with beans Compleats Homestyle	2.8%
Cooksimple Tamale Pie	2.9%
Old el Paso Cheesy Mexican Rice	2.9%

Boxed Meals - by sugar content (continued)

Meal	% Sugar
Pasta Roni Garlic & olive oil vermicelli	2.9%
Rice-a-Roni Chicken & mushroom Rice & Vermicelli mix	2.9%
Sam Mills Cheddar broccoli Gluten Free Pasta Sides	2.9%
Sam Mills White mac & cheese Deluxe	2.9%
Patel's Chickpea Curry	2.9%
Great Value Cheddar Broccoli & Rice	2.9%
Mrs Cubbison's Seasoned dressing	2.9%
Sam Mills Chicken Gluten Free Pasta Sides	2.9%
Zatarain's White cheddar chipotle Pasta dinner	2.9%
Sam Mills Beef Stroganoff	3.0%
Sam Mills Butter & herb Gluten Free Pasta Sides	3.0%
Tuna Helper Fettucini Alfredo	3.0%

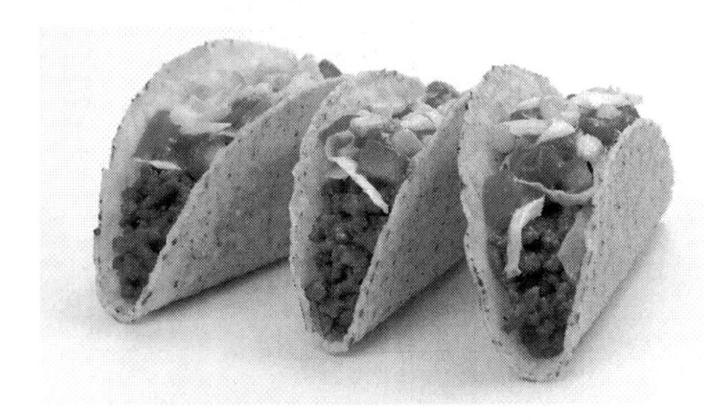

Boxed Meals - alphabetical

Brand	Item	Sub-Item	% Sugar
A Taste of Thai	Coconut Ginger Noodles		1.8%
Annie's Homegrown	Creamy Deluxe	Rice Pasta & Extra Cheesy Cheddar	1.9%
	Creamy Deluxe	Elbows & Four Cheese	2.1%
	Creamy Deluxe	Macaroni	2.2%
Augason Farms	72 Hour 1 person Emergency Kit		2.3%
Banquet	Homestyle Bakes	Cheesy Ham & Hash Brown	1.0%
	Homestyle Bakes	Dumplings & Chicken	1.6%
	Homestyle Bakes	Creamy Turkey & Stuffing	1.6%
	Homestyle Bakes	Chicken, Mashed Potato and Biscuits	1.7%
	Homestyle Bakes	Creamy Cheesy Chicken Alfredo	2.2%
	Homestyle Bakes	Biscuits & Chicken	2.5%
	Homestyle Bakes	Sausage Gravy & Biscuits	2.5%
Barilla	Tortellini	Three Cheese	1.8%
	Italian Entrees	Marinara Penne	2.7%
Betty Crocker	Mashed Potatoes	Creamy Butter	0.0%
	Mashed Potatoes	Riasted Garlic	0.0%
	Scalloped Potatoes		0.0%
	Helper Complete Meals	Chicken with Cheesy Rice & Broccoli	0.6%
	Helper Complete Meals	Fried Rice with Chicken	1.2%
	Helper Complete Meals	Cheesy Chicken	1.8%

Boxed Meals - alphabetical (continued)

Brand	Item	Sub-Item	% Sugar
Betty Crocker	Helper Complete Meals	Cheesy Beef taco	1.8%
	Helper Complete Meals	Chicken & Buttermilk Biscuits	1.8%
	Helper Complete Meals	Stroganoff	1.8%
	Helper Complete Meals	Chicken Fettuccine Alfredo	1.8%
Birds Eye	Steamfresh	Lightly sauced roasted red potatoes and green beans	1.9%
Conchita	Rice	Extra Fancy Long Grain	0.0%
	Rice	Long Grain Brown	0.0%
	Rice	Parboiled Long Grain	0.0%
Cooksimple	Tamale Pie		2.9%
Cugino's	Pasta Sides	Creamy Roasted Red Pepper	1.6%
	Pasta Sides	Mushroom Stroganoff	1.7%
Dinty Moore	Beef Stew		1.1%
Domo	Risotto	Four Cheese	1.8%
	Risotto	Mushrooms	1.8%
Fiesta	Round Duros		0.0%
Gillian's	Home-style Stuffing	Wheat and gluten free	0.0%
Gourmantra	Indian Meal Kit	Tandoori	0.0%
Goya	Mexican Rice	Chicken	2.2%
Great Value	Potatoes	Au Gratin	0.0%
	Instant Mashed Potatoes	Creamy Butter	0.0%

Boxed Meals - alphabetical (continued)

Brand	Item	Sub-Item	% Sugar
Great Value	Mashed Potatoes		0.0%
	Cheddar Broccoli & Rice		2.9%
Hamburger Helper	Crunchy Taco		2.4%
Healthy Choices	Modern Classics	Beef & Broccoli	1.6%
	Modern Classics	Herb Crusted Fish	2.6%
Heritage Select	Basmati	Roasted Chicken and Herb	2.2%
	Basmati	Roasted Garlic and Herb	2.2%
Hidden Valley	Pasta Salad	Original Ranch	2.5%
	Pasta Salad	Southwest Ranch	2.6%
Hormel	Compleats	Smoky bacon parmesan rigatoni	0.0%
	Compleats Homestyle	Chicken Breast & mashed potato	0.0%
	Compleats	Italian herb & cheese rigatoni	0.4%
	Compleats	Roast beef & gravy with mashed potatoes	0.4%
	Compleats	Salisbury steak with sliced potatoes & gravy	0.4%
	Compleats Homestyle	Macaroni & cheese	0.4%
	Compleats	Three cheese chicken pasta	0.4%
	Compleats Good Mornings	Bacon breakfast scramble	0.5%
	Compleats	Chicken & rice	0.7%

Boxed Meals - alphabetical (continued)

Brand	Item	Sub-Item	% Sugar
Hormel	Compleats Good Mornings	Sausage breakfast scramble	0.9%
	Microwave Bowls	Chicken & Dumplings	1.1%
	Compleats Homestyle	Beef Pot Roast	1.1%
	Compleats Homestyle	Chicken Breast & Dressing	1.1%
	Compleats Homestyle	Meatloaf & mashed potatoes	1.1%
	Compleats	Creamy Cheese & Basil tortellini	1.2%
	Compleats Good Mornings	Sausage Gravy & roasted potatoes	1.4%
	Country Crock	Cheesy diced potatoes	1.4%
	Compleats	Beef Steak & Peppers	1.4%
	Compleats	Chicken Pasta Primavera	1.4%
	Compleats	Turkey & dressing with gravy	1.4%
	Compleats	Spaghetti & turkey meatballs	1.8%
	Compleats	Cheese & Spinach	2.5%
	Compleats Homestyle	Chilli with beans	2.8%
Hungry Jack	Mashed Potatoes	Naturally flavoured	0.0%
Jyoti	Mung dal	with spinach	0.9%
	Channa dal	with zucchini	2.6%
Kartoffelland	Raw potato dumplings		0.0%
Kitchens of India	Curry	Rajma Masala red kidney beans	0.0%

Boxed Meals - alphabetical (continued)

Brand	Item	Sub-Item	% Sugar
Kitchens of India	Curry	Chickpea	0.8%
	Curry	Spinach palak paneer	0.8%
	Basmati rice pilaf	with vegetable & nuts	1.4%
	Basmati rice pilaf	with vegetables	2.1%
	Curry	Pav Bhaji mashed vegetable	2.4%
Knorr	Rice sides	Buffalo chicken rice	0.0%
	Rice sides	Steak fajitas rice	1.6%
	Rice sides	Rice pilaf	1.6%
	Pasta Sides	Chicken	1.7%
Kohinoor	Punjabi kadhi pakora		0.0%
	Dal palak with rice & curry		0.3%
	Madras lemon rice with sambhar		0.9%
	Mutter paneer		2.0%
Kraft	Velveeta Cheesy Skillets	Chicken Alfredo	2.0%
	Velveeta Cheesy Skillets	Chicken Chilli Cheese mac	2.0%
	Velveeta Cheesy Skillets	Lasagna with meat	2.4%
	Velveeta Cheesy Skillets	Ultimate Cheeseburger	2.4%
	Homestyle Macaroni & Cheese	Hearty Four Cheese	2.4%
La Choy	Creations	Asian fried rice	1.0%
La Tiara	Mexican taco shells		0.0%

Boxed Meals - alphabetical (continued)

Brand	Item	Sub-Item	% Sugar
Laurie's Kitchen	Chicken Parmesan truffle		2.2%
Louisiana	Cajun Etouffee Mix		0.0%
	Cajun Gumbo mix		0.0%
	Seasoned chicken fry		0.0%
	Dirty rice mix		2.2%
Louisiana Purchase	Jambalaya rice mix		1.8%
Luzianne	Jambalaya dinner kit		0.0%
Maggi	Spaetzle dumplings		2.2%
Marcy's	Traditional stuffing mix		0.0%
Margaret Holmes	Simple Suppers	Creole fixins	1.3%
McCormick	Rice	Paella	0.0%
	Rice	Chicken flavour	1.5%
Mrs Cubbison's	Seasoned dressing		2.9%
Mrs Leeper's	Creamy tuna & pasta mix		2.4%
Nalley	Tamales	Beef in chilli sauce	0.7%
Near East	Long grain and wild rice	Roasted vegetable & chicken	1.8%
	Rice pilaf mix	Toasted almond	1.8%
Nongshim	Noodle soup	Spicy Chicken	2.3%
Old el Paso	Tortilla stuffers	Carne Asada steak	1.8%
	Tortilla stuffers	Garlic Chili chicken	2.0%

Boxed Meals - alphabetical (continued)

Brand	Item	Sub-Item	% Sugar
Old el Paso	Taco dinner kit	Stand N Stuff	2.5%
	Cheesy Mexican Rice		2.9%
Osem	Mejadar rice & lentils		2.0%
	Meals on the go	Couscous & vegetables	2.4%
Pasta Roni	Garlic & olive oil vermicelli		2.9%
Patak's	Potato & spinach curry		0.4%
	Lentil curry		1.1%
	Butter chicken with rice		1.4%
	Chicken curry		1.8%
Patel's	Curry	Potato & Green pea	1.0%
	Basmati rice with green peas		1.4%
	Curry	Chickpea	2.9%
Ready Pac Foods	Bistro Chef Salad		2.3%
Rice-a-Roni	Rice pilaf		0.0%
	Rice & Vermicelli mix	Chicken	1.8%
	Rice & Vermicelli mix	Chicken teriyaki	1.8%
	Rice & Vermicelli mix	Chicken & mushroom	2.9%
Road's End Organics	Mac & cheese	Alfredo style	1.2%
	Penne & Cheese	Cheddar style	1.2%

Boxed Meals - alphabetical (continued)

Brand	Item	Sub-Item	% Sugar
Sam Miguel	White rice with vegetables	0.7%	
Sam Mills	Gluten Free Pasta Sides	Alfredo	2.8%
	Gluten Free Pasta Sides	Cheddar broccoli	2.9%
	Deluxe	White mac & cheese	2.9%
	Gluten Free Pasta Sides	Chicken	2.9%
	Beef Stroganoff		3.0%
	Gluten Free Pasta Sides	Butter & herb	3.0%
Side Mates	Original pearl couscous		2.0%
Slap Ya Mama	Cajun Jambalaya Mix		1.8%
	Cajun Red beans & rice		1.8%
Spam	Meal for 1	Spam & cheesy potatoes	1.4%
	Meal for 2	Spam & roasted potatoes with gravy	1.8%
	Meal for 3	Spam & scalloped potatoes	2.1%
St Dalfour	Gourmet on the go	Tuna & pasta	0.0%
	Gourmet on the go	Wild salmon with vegetables	0.0%
	Gourmet on the go	Three beans with sweetcorn	0.0%
SuperPretzel	Softstix	Cheese filled	2.0%
Taco Bell	Taco dinner kit	Crunchy & soft	1.7%
	Taco dinner kit	Crunchy	2.4%

Boxed Meals - alphabetical (continued)

Brand	Item	Sub-Item	% Sugar
Taste of Bombay	Chicken Tikka Masala		0.8%
Tasty Bite	Kashmir spinach		0.7%
	Aloo Palak		2.1%
	Bombay Potatoes		2.1%
	Jaipur Vegetables		2.1%
	Spinach channa		2.1%
	Peas Paneer		2.8%
	Vegetable Korma		2.8%
TGI Fridays	Chicken wings	Buffalo style sauce	0.0%
Thai Kitchen	Stir-fry rice noodles		0.0%
Tony Chachere's	Creole yellow rice		2.2%
	Dry Creole	Dirty rice	2.2%
	Dry Creole	Jambalaya dinner mix	2.6%
Truly Indian	Chatpate Choley		0.0%
	Matar paneer		0.0%
TruRoots	Pilaf	Curry rice multigrain	1.0%
	Pilaf	Mediterranean vegetable multigrain	2.8%
Tuna Helper	Fettucini Alfredo		3.0%
Udon	Noodles	Mushroom	1.0%
Uncle Ben's	Ready Rice	Teriyaki	1.3%
Vigo	Yellow rice & seafood dinner		1.1%
	Long grain white & wild rice		1.8%

Boxed Meals - alphabetical (continued)

Brand	Item	Sub-Item	% Sugar
	Seasoned risotto with broccoli		1.8%
Weight Watchers	Smart Ones	Three cheese omelette	1.2%
Zatarain's	Big Easy rice	Dirty	0.0%
	Big Easy rice	Jambalaya	0.0%
	Big Easy rice	Red rice & beans	0.0%
	Gumbo mix		0.0%
	New Orleans Style	Dirty brown rice	0.0%
	New Orleans Style	Etouffee base	0.0%
	New Orleans Style	Original dirty rice	0.0%
	New Orleans Style	Original Jambalaya rice	0.0%
	Big Easy rice	Garden vegetable brown rice	1.4%
	New Orleans Style	Red beans & rice	1.8%
	Wild brown rice		1.8%
	New Orleans Style	Brown rice jambalaya mix	2.5%
	New Orleans Style	Jambalaya pasta dinner	2.6%
	New Orleans Style	Spanish rice	2.7%
	Pasta dinner	Southern stroganoff	2.7%
	Pasta dinner	White cheddar chipotle	2.9%
Ziyad	Pilaf	Roasted Green wheat	0.0%
	Pilaf	Rice & lentil	0.0%

Fast Food

Supermarkets aren't the only place you'll be buying food prepared by others. To cover off the majority of the market for 'restaurant' food, in this section, I've analysed the menu's of the major fast food chains.

WARNING: All fried food sold in these restaurants in the USA has been fried in seed oils and should be avoided if you are concerned about seed oils.

Subway Restaurants

Menu Item	% Sugar
Condiments Chipotle Southwest	0.0%
Condiments Light Mayonnaise	0.0%
Condiments Mayonnaise	0.0%
Condiments Mustard	0.0%
Condiments Olive Oil Blend	0.0%
Condiments Vinegar	0.0%
Extra Toppings Bacon Strip	0.0%
Extra Toppings Cheese Triangle Cheddar	0.0%
Extra Toppings Cheese Triangle Pepperjack	0.0%
Extra Toppings Cheese Triangle Processed American	0.0%
Extra Toppings Cheese Triangle Provolone	0.0%
Extra Toppings Cheese Triangle Swiss	0.0%
Extra Toppings Cheese Triangle Monterey	0.0%
Bread Wrap	0.0%

Subway Restaurants (continued)

Menu Item	% Sugar
All Day Soup Chicken Noodle	0.4%
Breakfast Egg White 3" Flatbread Bacon, Egg & Cheese with Avocado	0.9%
Breakfast Egg White 3" Flatbread Egg with Cheese & Avocado	0.9%
Breakfast Egg White 3" Flatbread Steak, Egg & Cheese	0.9%
All Day Salads Double Chicken Salad	0.9%
Breakfast Egg White 3" Flatbread Black Forrest Ham, Egg & Cheese	1.0%
All Day Salads Big Hot Pastrami Melt Salad	1.0%
Breakfast Egg White 3" Flatbread Bacon, Egg & Cheese	1.0%
Breakfast Egg White 3" Flatbread Egg & Cheese	1.1%
All Day Salads Oven Roasted Chicken Salad	1.1%
All Day Soup Clam Chowder	1.2%
All Day Soup Creamy Chicken Dumplings	1.2%
All Day Soup Vegetable Beef	1.2%
All Day Salads Turkey & Bacon With Avocado Salad	1.2%
All Day Salads Turkey Jalapeno Melt Salad	1.3%
Breakfast Egg White 3" Flatbread Sunrise Subway Melt	1.4%
All Day Salads Subway Club Salad	1.4%
All Day Salads Veggie Delite Salad	1.4%
All Day Salads Roast Beef Salad	1.4%
All Day Salads Big Philly Cheesesteak Salad	1.4%
All Day Salads Subway Club With Avocado Salad	1.5%
All Day Salads Turkey Breast & Ham Salad	1.5%
All Day Salads Turkey Breast Salad	1.5%
All Day Salads Steak & Bacon Melt Salad	1.5%

Subway Restaurants (continued)

Menu Item	% Sugar
All Day Soup Creamy Wild and Brown Rice	1.6%
All Day Soup Loaded Baked Potato	1.6%
All Day Soup Minestrone	1.6%
All Day Salads Chipotle Chicken & Cheese Salad	1.6%
All Day Salads Chipotle Steak & Cheese Salad	1.6%
All Day Salads BBQ Steak & Bacon Melt Salad	1.6%
Breakfast Egg White 3" Flatbread Breakfast B.M.T. Melt	1.7%
Breakfast Regular Egg on 3" Flatbread Breakfast B.M.T. Melt	1.7%
All Day Salads Black Forest Ham Salad	1.8%
Breakfast Regular Egg on 3" Flatbread Bacon, Egg & Cheese with Avocado	1.8%
All Day Salads Sriracha Chicken Melt Salad	1.8%
All Day Salads Fritos Chicken Enchilada Melt Salad	1.8%
All Day Salads Spicy Tuna Salad	1.8%
Breakfast Regular Egg on 3" Flatbread Steak, Egg & Cheese	1.9%
Breakfast Regular Egg on 3" Flatbread Black Forrest Ham, Egg & Cheese	1.9%
All Day Flatizza Cheese	1.9%
All Day Soup Green Chili and Tomato	2.0%
All Day Salads Sriracha Steak Melt Salad	2.0%
Breakfast Regular Egg on 3" Flatbread Sunrise Subway Melt	2.0%
Breakfast Regular Egg on 3" Flatbread Bacon, Egg & Cheese	2.1%
All Day Flatizza Veggie	2.1%
Breakfast Regular Egg on 3" Flatbread Egg & Cheese	2.2%
All Day Flatizza Pepperoni	2.2%
All Day Flatizza Spicy Italian	2.2%

Subway Restaurants (continued)

Menu Item	% Sugar
Breakfast Egg White Omelet 6" Sandwich Bacon, Egg & Cheese with Avocado	2.3%
Bread 6" Flatbread	2.3%
All Day Soup Golden Broccoli and Cheese	2.4%
Breakfast Egg White Omelet 6" Sandwich Egg with Cheese & Avocado	2.4%
All Day 6" Sandwich Big Hot Pastrami	2.5%
All Day 6" Sandwich Tuna	2.6%
Breakfast Egg White Omelet 6" Sandwich Sunrise Subway Melt	2.6%
Breakfast Egg White Omelet 6" Sandwich Breakfast B.M.T. Melt	2.7%
All Day 6" Sandwich Turkey & Bacon Avocado	2.7%
All Day 6" Sandwich Turkey Jalapeno Melt	2.7%
All Day 6" Sandwich Big Philly Cheesesteak	2.7%
Breakfast Egg White Omelet 6" Sandwich Bacon, Egg & Cheese	2.7%
All Day Soup Beef Chili	2.7%
All Day Soup Chili Con Carne	2.7%
All Day Soup Poblano Corn Chowder	2.7%
All Day 6" Sandwich Chicken & Bacon Ranch Melt	2.8%
Breakfast Egg White Omelet 6" Sandwich Steak, Egg & Cheese	2.8%
Breakfast Egg White Omelet 6" Sandwich Western, Egg & Cheese	2.8%
Breakfast Egg White Omelet 6" Sandwich Egg & Cheese	2.9%
Breakfast Omelet 6" Sandwich Sunrise Subway Melt	2.9%
All Day 6" Sandwich Subway Club	3.0%
Breakfast Egg White Omelet 6" Sandwich Egg & Cheese with Ham	3.0%

McDonald's

All items are without dipping sauce. Anything fried has been fried in a seed oil.

Menu Item	% Sugar
Hash Brown	0.0%
10 Piece Chicken McNuggets	0.0%
Kids Fries	0.0%
Large Fries	0.0%
Medium Fries	0.0%
Small Fries	0.0%
Classic Large Big Breakfast	1.1%
Egg White Regular Big Breakfast	1.1%
Classic Regular Big Breakfast	1.1%
Sausage with Egg Regular Biscuit	1.2%
Sausage With Egg McMuffin	1.3%
Sausage With Egg White McMuffin	1.3%
Egg White Large Big Breakfast	1.4%
Steak, Egg & Cheese Regular Biscuit	1.5%
Chicken & Bacon Grilled Premium McWrap	1.6%
Steak, Egg & Cheese McMuffin	1.6%
Sausage with Egg White Large Biscuit	1.7%
Sausage with Egg Large Biscuit	1.7%
Ranch Grilled Snack Wrap	1.7%
Sausage Regular Biscuit	1.7%

McDonalds (continued)

Menu Item	% Sugar
Honey Mustard Grilled Snack Wrap	1.7%
Sausage with Egg White Regular Biscuit	1.8%
Sausage Burrito	1.8%
Sausage McMuffin	1.8%
Steak, Egg & Cheese Large Biscuit	1.9%
Chicken & Ranch Grilled Premium McWrap	1.9%
Bacon, Egg White & Cheese Regular Biscuit	2.0%
Bacon, Egg & Cheese Regular Biscuit	2.0%
Southern Style Chicken Regular Biscuit	2.1%
Egg McMuffin	2.2%
Chicken & Bacon Crispy Premium McWrap	2.2%
Egg White Delight McMuffin	2.2%
Sausage Large Biscuit	2.3%
Bacon, Egg White & Cheese Large Biscuit	2.4%
Mac Snack Wrap	2.4%
Ranch Crispy Snack Wrap	2.4%
Bacon, Egg & Cheese Large Biscuit	2.4%
Honey Mustard Crispy Snack Wrap	2.4%
Chicken & Ranch Crispy Premium McWrap	2.5%
Southern Style Chicken Large Biscuit	2.5%
Bacon Ranch With Grilled Chicken Premium Salad	2.6%
Steak, Egg & Cheese Bagel	2.9%

Burger King

All items are without dipping sauce. Anything fried has been fried in a seed oil.

Menu Item	% Sugar
Value French Fries	0.0%
Small French Fries	0.0%
Medium French Fries	0.0%
Large French Fries	0.0%
Value Satisfries French Fries	0.0%
Small Satisfries French Fries	0.0%
Medium Satisfries French Fries	0.0%
Large Satisfries French Fries	0.0%
Home-style Chicken Strip	0.0%
Buffalo Chicken Strip	0.0%
Chicken Nugget	0.0%
Hash Brown	0.0%
Crispy Ranch Chicken Wrap	0.7%
Grilled Ranch Chicken Wrap	0.7%
Original Quaker Oatmeal	0.8%
Avocado Ranch Dressing Side Garden Salad	1.2%
Tendergrill Chicken BLT Garden Fresh Salad	1.4%
Grilled Chicken BLT Garden Fresh Salad	1.6%
Sausage & Cheese BK Breakfast Muffin Sandwich	1.6%
Sausage Breakfast Burrito	1.6%

Burger King (continued)

Menu Item	% Sugar
Southwestern Breakfast Burrito	1.7%
Tendergrill Chicken Caesar Garden Fresh Salad	1.7%
Grilled Chicken Caesar Garden Fresh Salad	1.7%
Sausage, Egg & Cheese BK Breakfast Muffin Sandwich	1.8%
Crispy Chicken BLT Garden Fresh Salad	2.0%
Tendercrisp Chicken BLT Garden Fresh Salad	2.1%
Crispy Chicken Caesar Garden Fresh Salad	2.1%
Tendercrisp Chicken Caesar Garden Fresh Salad	2.1%
Sausage, Egg & Cheese Biscuit	2.1%
Country Ham & Egg Biscuit	2.2%
Bacon, Egg & Cheese BK Breakfast Muffin Sandwich	2.3%
Mozzarella Stick	2.3%
Sausage Biscuit	2.4%
Egg & Cheese BK Breakfast Muffin Sandwich	2.4%
Bacon, Egg & Cheese Biscuit	2.5%
Ham, Egg & Cheese BK Breakfast Muffin Sandwich	2.5%
Sausage, Egg & Cheese Double Croissan'wich	2.6%
Side Caesar Salad	2.6%
Triple Whopper	2.6%
Crispy Chicken Jr.	2.8%
Tendergrill Chicken Sandwich	2.9%

Pizza Hut

Note: These figures have not been adjusted for lactose (in the cheese) content as it is difficult to accurately estimate. All figures would be lower when adjusted for lactose. All these are without dipping sauce unless it says otherwise.

Menu Item	% Sugar
All American Traditional Bone-In Wings	0.0%
All American Crispy Bone-In Wings	0.0%
Hot Baked Wings Wings	0.0%
Mild Baked Wings Wings	0.0%
Wedge Fries Sides	0.0%
Diet Pepsi Medium Drinks	0.0%
5 Cheese Please Garlic Parmesan Base Pizza	0.4%
Roasted Veggie Garlic Parmesan Base Pizza	0.5%
Super Supreme Hand Tossed Style Pizza	0.9%
Supreme Hand Tossed Style Pizza	1.0%
Meat Lovers Hand Tossed Style Pizza	1.0%
Chicken Supreme Hand Tossed Style Pizza	1.0%
Veggie Lovers Hand Tossed Style Pizza	1.0%
Chicken Alfredo Pasta	1.1%
Meaty P-Zone Pizza	1.1%
Pepperoni Lovers Hand Tossed Style Pizza	1.1%
Cheese Only Hand Tossed Style Pizza	1.2%
Pepperoni Hand Tossed Style Pizza	1.3%
Ultimate Cheese Lovers Hand Tossed Style Pizza	1.3%
Pepperoni P-Zone Pizza	1.3%
Garlic Parmesan Crispy Bone-In Wings	1.4%
Garlic Parmesan Bone-Out Wings	1.4%

Pizza Hut (continued)

Menu Item	% Sugar
Classic P-Zone Pizza	1.7%
Garlic Parmesan Traditional Bone-In Wings	1.8%
Chicken, Bacon, Tomato Garlic Parmesan Base Pizza	1.8%
Meat Lovers Pan Pizza	1.8%
All American Bone-Out Wings	1.9%
Pepperoni Lovers Pan Pizza	2.0%
Cheese Only Pan Pizza	2.2%
Pepperoni Pan Pizza	2.2%
Ultimate Cheese Lovers Pan Pizza	2.3%
Ranch Dipping Sauce Wings	2.3%
Super Supreme Pan Pizza	2.5%
Fried Cheese Sticks Sides	2.5%
Stuffed Pizza Rollers Sides	2.6%
Buffalo Mild Crispy Bone-In Wings	2.7%
Buffalo Medium Crispy Bone-In Wings	2.7%
Buffalo Burnin Hot Crispy Bone-In Wings	2.7%
Supreme Pan Pizza	2.7%
Buffalo Mild Bone-Out Wings	2.7%
Buffalo Medium Bone-Out Wings	2.7%
Buffalo Burnin Hot Bone-Out Wings	2.7%
Chicken Supreme Pan Pizza	2.8%
Meaty Marinara Pasta	2.9%

KFC

All items are without dipping sauce. Anything fried has been fried in a seed oil.

Menu Item	% Sugar
Original Recipe Thigh Chicken	0.0%
Extra Crispy Thigh Chicken	0.0%
Spicy Crispy Thigh Chicken	0.0%
Kentucky Grilled Thigh Chicken	0.0%
Extra Crispy Tenders Strips	0.0%
Original Recipe Bites	0.0%
Hot Wings	0.0%
Fiery Buffalo Hot Wings	0.0%
Original Recipe Bites Snack Box	0.0%
Extra Crispy Boneless Piece Go Cup	0.0%
Extra Crispy Tenders Go Cup	0.0%
Original Recipe Bites Go Cup	0.0%
Hot Wings Go Cup	0.0%
Fiery Buffalo Hot Wings Go Cup	0.0%
Hot Wings Value Box	0.0%
Fiery Buffalo Hot Wings Value Box	0.0%
Grilled Value Box	0.0%
Original Recipe Value Box	0.0%
Extra Crispy Value Box	0.0%
Mashed Potatoes with Gravy	0.0%
Mashed Potatoes without Gravy	0.0%
Gravy with Bites	0.0%
Potato Wedges	0.0%
Gizzards	0.0%
Livers	0.0%

KFC (continued)

Menu Item	% Sugar
Country Fried Steak with Peppered White Gravy	0.0%
Country Fried Steak without Peppered White Gravy	0.0%
Jalapeno Peppers	0.0%
Buttery Spread	0.0%
Sauce Cup Creamy Buffalo	0.0%
Snack Size Famous Bowls	0.5%
Potato & Gravy Famous Bowls	0.6%
Hot Shots Bites	0.8%
Crispy Chicken Caesar Without Dressing or Croutons Salads	1.0%
Caesar Without Dressing or Croutons Salads	1.1%
Green Beans	1.2%
Crispy Chicken BLT Without Dressing or Croutons Salads	1.4%
Macaroni & Cheese	1.5%
Crispy Twister Sandwiches	1.7%
House Without Dressing or Croutons Salads	1.9%
Chicken Little Go Cup	1.9%

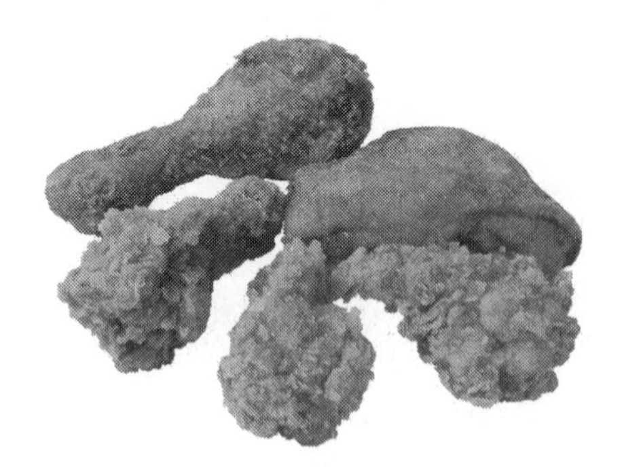

Taco Bell

All items are without dipping sauce. Anything fried has been fried in a seed oil.

Menu Item	% Sugar
Hash Brown	0.0%
Avocado Ranch Dressing	0.0%
Fire Border Sauce	0.0%
Hot Border Sauce	0.0%
Mild Border Sauce	0.0%
Cilantro Dressing	0.0%
Guacamole	0.0%
Pepper Jack Sauce	0.0%
Red Sauce	0.0%
Salsa Verde	0.0%
Premium Latin Rice	0.0%
Tostada	0.6%
Black Beans and Rice	0.7%
Cheesy Fiesta Potatoes	0.8%
Pintos n Cheese	0.8%
Chips and Guacamole	0.9%
Chicken Cantina Bowl	1.0%
Steak Cantina Bowl	1.0%
Veggie Cantina Bowl	1.0%
Crispy Potato Soft Taco	1.0%
Beef Smothered Burrito	1.0%
Shredded Chicken Smothered Burrito	1.0%

Taco Bell (continued)

Menu Item	% Sugar
Steak Smothered Burrito	1.0%
Fresco Crunchy Taco	1.1%
Beef Soft Taco	1.1%
Chicken Soft Taco	1.1%
Steak and Egg Breakfast Burrito	1.2%
Steak and Egg Burrito	1.2%
Spicy Chicken Cool Ranch DLT	1.2%
Sausage Breakfast Burrito	1.2%
Express Taco Salad with Chips	1.3%
Steak A.M. Crunchwrap	1.3%
Bacon A.M. Grilled Taco	1.3%
Sausage A.M. Grilled Taco	1.3%
Chicken Cool Ranch DLT	1.3%
Cool Ranch Doritos Locos Taco	1.3%
Crunchy Taco	1.3%
Fiery Doritos Locos Taco	1.3%
Nacho Cheese Doritos Locos Taco	1.3%
Combo Burrito	1.3%
Chili Cheese Burrito	1.3%
Double Decker Taco	1.3%
Sausage A.M. Crunchwrap	1.4%
Chicken XXL Grilled Stuft Burrito	1.4%
Steak XXL Grilled Stuft Burrito	1.4%
Mexican Pizza	1.4%

Taco Bell (continued)

Menu Item	% Sugar
Bacon A.M. Crunchwrap	1.4%
Black Bean Burrito	1.5%
Beef Fiesta Taco Salad	1.5%
Chicken Fiesta Taco Salad	1.5%
Steak Fiesta Taco Salad	1.5%
Egg and Cheese A.M. Grilled Taco	1.6%
Chicken Cantina Burrito	1.6%
Steak Cantina Burrito	1.6%
Bean Burrito	1.6%
Beef XXL Grilled Stuft Burrito	1.6%
Black Beans	1.6%
Nachos BellGrande	1.6%
Supreme Double Decker Taco	1.6%
Chicken Quesadilla	1.7%
Steak Quesadilla	1.7%
Beef Burrito Supreme	1.7%
Chicken Burrito Supreme	1.7%
Steak Burrito Supreme	1.7%
MexiMelt	1.7%
Fresco Grilled Steak Soft Taco	1.7%
Cheesy Potato Burrito	1.7%
7-Layer Burrito	1.7%
Chicken Fresco Burrito Supreme	1.7%
Steak Fresco Burrito Supreme	1.7%

Taco Bell (continued)

Menu Item	% Sugar
Cheese Roll-Up	1.8%
Supreme Crunchy Taco	1.8%
Supreme Fiery Doritos Locos Taco	1.8%
Supreme Nacho Cheese Doritos Locos Taco	1.8%
Chicken Burrito	1.8%
Grilled Steak Soft Taco	1.8%
Bacon Breakfast Burrito	1.8%
Fresco Style Bacon Breakfast Burrito	1.9%
Fresco Style Sausage Breakfast Burrito	1.9%
Fresco Style Steak and Egg Breakfast Burrito	1.9%
Veggie Cantina Burrito	1.9%
Chips and Pico De Gallo	1.9%
Chili Cheese Fries Loaded Griller	1.9%
Fresco Soft Taco	1.9%
Fresco Chicken Soft Taco	1.9%
Beefy Nacho Griller	1.9%
Quesarito	1.9%
Nachos	2.0%
Nachos Supreme	2.0%
Chipotle Ranch Chicken Loaded Griller	2.1%
Cheese Quesadilla	2.2%
Beefy 5-Layer Burrito	2.2%
Loaded Potato Griller	2.3%
Crunchwrap Supreme	2.3%

Taco Bell (continued)

Menu Item	% Sugar
Cheesy Gordita Crunch	2.3%
Supreme Beef Soft Taco	2.3%
Cheesy Nachos	2.4%
Supreme Spicy Chicken Cool Ranch DLT	2.5%
Chicken Chalupa Supreme	2.6%
Steak Chalupa Supreme	2.6%
Veggie Chalupa Supreme	2.6%
Supreme Chicken Cool Ranch DLT	2.7%
Supreme Cool Ranch Doritos Locos Taco	2.7%

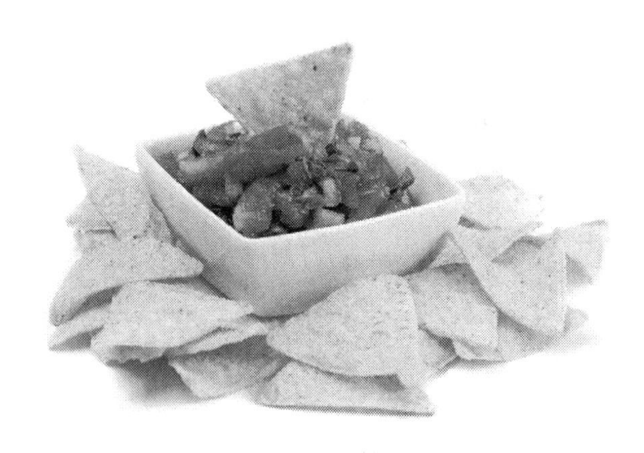

More Information

Still haven't found what you're looking for? I also maintain a database of over 2,000 foods including restaurant meals typically found in Asian and Mediterranean restaurants.

You can search the database for free at www.davidgillespie.org

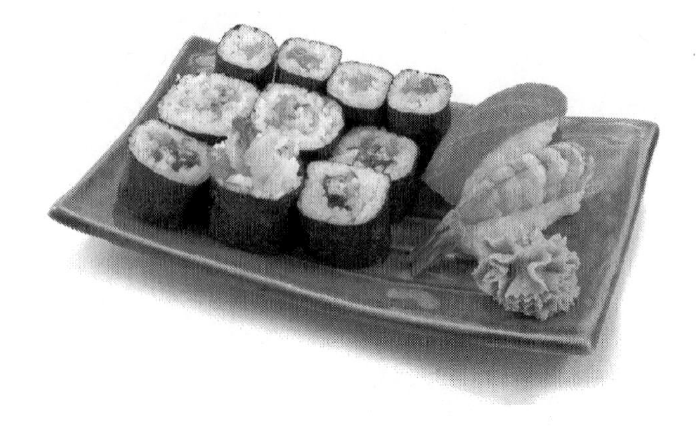